Becoming a
HEALTHCARE
PROFESSIONAL

DATE DUE

NOV 23	

DEMCO, INC. 38-2931

Related Titles

Becoming a Nurse
Dental Assisting Exam
Health Occupations Entrance Exam
Medical Assistant: Preparation for the CMA and RMA Exams
Nursing Assistant/Nurse's Aide Exam
Physical Therapist Assistant Exam

Becoming a

HEALTHCARE

PROFESSIONAL

LEARNINGEXPRESS®

New York

Library of Congress Cataloging-in-Publication Data:
Becoming a healthcare professional.
   p. ; cm.
  ISBN: 978-1-57685-729-8
  1. Allied health personnel—Vocational guidance.   I. LearningExpress (Organization)
  [DNLM: 1. Allied Health Personnel.   2. Career Choice.   3. Vocational Guidance.
W 21.5 B398 2010]
  R697.A4B427   2010
  610.73'7069023—dc22

                                                                              2009043244

Printed in the United States of America

9 8 7 6 5 4 3 2 1

ISBN 978-1-57685-729-8

For more information or to place an order, contact LearningExpress at:
  2 Rector Street
  26th Floor
  New York, NY 10006

Or visit us at:
  www.learnatest.com

Contents

Introduction

Why Enter the Healthcare Field?

THE HEALTHCARE industry is one of the fastest-growing segments in the U.S. economy. The U.S. Department of Labor calls healthcare an "industry supersector" that is expected to contribute to an 18.8% growth and the addition of more jobs than *any* other industry through 2016. In fact, healthcare and social assistance—including public and private hospitals, nursing and residential care facilities, and individual and family services—will add 4 million new jobs, thanks to increased demands because of an aging population and longer life expectancies.

According to the U.S. Department of Labor, healthcare support occupations are expected to grow at 26.8%, the fastest among all support occupations. The fastest growing healthcare industry support occupation jobs, by degree or educational requirements, are:

associate degree: includes cardiovascular technologist and technician, dental hygienist, and physical therapy assistant

postsecondary vocational award: includes nursing aide, orderly, and attendant.

In addition to robust job growth, there are many other exciting reasons to pursue a career in healthcare. Because healthcare costs have risen steadily over the last decade, the healthcare industry has changed to become more cost conscious. Employees are being given more responsibility earlier in their careers. This means that many of the new jobs in the healthcare field will be filled by employees with two years of training or less, and these employees will be more involved in direct patient care than in the past.

Along with increased cost consciousness, the healthcare market is changing as new medicine and technology alter the ways in which patients are treated. Such innovations as anesthesia that wears off quickly, outpatient rehabilitation units, and less invasive surgical procedures mean that the length of patients' hospital stays are reduced. In general, there is a movement away from hospital care to outpatient services and home care. This trend contributes to the job opportunities for employees with two years of training or less. These trends do not mean that the quality of care is diminished. In fact, the move away from hospital care to home care can be a very positive trend for many patients, particularly the elderly, who may be more comfortable receiving care in their own homes.

Another important result of the increased demand for healthcare workers is improved earning potential. The average earnings for nonsupervisory workers in healthcare are higher than the average for all private industries. Hospital workers, who make up the largest pool of all healthcare workers, earn substantially more on average. (Even though there is movement away from hospital care, hospitals will continue to be the largest employers of healthcare workers.) With the increased demand for healthcare workers in the years ahead, the earning potential will only get better.

This book focuses on the following entry-level positions with high growth potential: **dental assistant, medical assistant, nursing assistant, physical therapy assistant, radiologic technician,** and **surgical technician**. The wealth of jobs available makes any of these positions a possibility for your future.

Some people want to enter the healthcare field in one area and then seek additional training for more advanced positions, and others are happy to stay in their original position. The healthcare field offers you the flexibility to make such decisions because both alternatives are within reach.

In this book you will learn all about getting started in this exciting field. In Chapter 1, you will discover the hottest careers in the field that require a maximum of two years of training. Chapter 2 gives you details about getting the training you need to pursue your new career. Chapter 3 contains a directory of training programs for you to explore. Chapter 4 provides a wealth of information about financing your training. Chapter 5 offers important strategies for finding job opportunities and will help you land the job of your choice by showing you how to write a convincing cover letter and resume and make a great impression in an interview. Chapter 6, you will learn how to succeed in your new career, with special tips for meeting the challenges of healthcare work.

This is a step-by-step guide to starting a career in healthcare from deciding on a field to getting training and from finding and winning a job to succeeding and getting ahead. In the back of the book, you will find a wealth of resources that will point you to organizations and websites that can help you get your career started, achieve your training goals, and support you throughout your career.

There has never been a better time to enter the healthcare field. Even beyond the job opportunities and earning potential, healthcare is a career that offers tremendous job satisfaction because it is devoted to helping others and provides a vital service in the community. Now is also a time of great innovation in the field. Doctors and researchers are continually making discoveries and advancements that are improving the quality of care and overall life expectancy. Read on to learn more about the important and exciting careers in the healthcare field and the inside information you need to succeed.

CHAPTER one

THE HOTTEST HEALTHCARE JOBS AND HOW TO GET THEM

THIS CHAPTER describes the most exciting and lucrative entry-level healthcare jobs that require only two years of training or less, so that you can begin your career in healthcare as quickly as possible. It includes specific job descriptions, typical salaries, advancement opportunities, hiring trends, and the skills needed for each job. You'll learn about different types of employers and their typical hiring procedures, including alternatives to hospital work. You'll also find inside advice from healthcare workers.

DENTAL ASSISTANT

Dental assistants perform a variety of patient care, administrative, and laboratory duties in dentists' offices, including the tasks listed below.

- ▶ They may work chairside, preparing patients for treatment and offering the materials and tools the dentist needs to examine and treat patients.
- ▶ They make patients as comfortable as possible in the dental chair, using a suction hose to keep the patient's mouth dry and clear, explaining procedures, and performing tooth cleanings.

▶ They may remove sutures, apply anesthetics and cavity-preventive agents to teeth and gums, remove cement used in the filling process, and place dental dams on the teeth to isolate them for individual treatment.

▶ They also sterilize and disinfect instruments and equipment, prepare tray setups for dental procedures, provide postoperative instruction, and instruct patients on oral healthcare.

▶ They may operate x-ray machines and develop x-rays.

▶ If they have laboratory duties, they make casts of teeth and mouth from impressions taken by dentists, and make temporary crowns.

▶ They may have administrative duties such as scheduling appointments, receiving patients, keeping treatment records, sending bills, receiving payments, and ordering supplies.

Typical Salaries

On average, dental assistants earn $24,000 to $33,000 or more annually working full time, depending on the amount of training they have received. When they gain more experience, they earn higher salaries.

Typical Salaries for Dental Assistants in Different Areas

City	Low End	Average	High End
Charlotte, NC	26,130	32,177	38,334
El Paso, TX	23,135	28,833	33,941
Jacksonville, FL	25,106	31,034	36,833
Los Angeles, CA	29,704	34,169	43,579
Milwaukee, WI	27,854	34,103	40,864
New York, NY	31,376	38,706	46,031
San Francisco, CA	32,111	39,856	47,110

Source: www.swz.salary.com

Hiring Trends

Most dental assistants work with group or private practices; some work in dental schools, government hospitals, public health departments, and clinics.

Employment opportunities for dental assistants are expected to grow much faster than average through the year 2012. As the population continues to grow, so does general awareness of the importance of dental health. Dental insurance is expected to become available to more people, which means more people will use dental services and will retain their natural teeth later in life. All of these factors add up to increased patient loads for dentist, and they will need to rely on support personnel such as dental hygienists and assistants to help deliver quality care for all patients. Additional job openings will arise when assistants leave the occupation or decide to further their education.

Personal Abilities and Personality Traits Needed

Cleanliness is a priority in a dental office, and dentists expect their assistants to be clean, neat, and well-groomed at all times.

Dentists look for assistants who have good people skills. Dental assistants work with many kinds of people, including children and the elderly. Some patients are anxious about receiving dental care, so dental assistants need to be friendly and empathetic in order to help put patients at ease.

Manual dexterity is another important skill for dental assistants. They need to be able to handle instruments carefully and quickly.

Dentists look for assistants who are reliable. The work is sometimes routine, and dental assistants need to be able to maintain a positive, professional attitude regardless of the work they are doing.

Computers are commonplace in dental practices, and computer skills have become important for dental assistants. Many dentists keep electronic patient records and treatment plans and many dental assistants use computers chairside to review patient treatment plans, view x-ray images, schedule appointments, and show oral care tutorials to patients. Dental assistants who are proficient with spreadsheets, text documents, electronic calendars, and email will have a competitive edge in finding employment.

Dental assistants may be expected to work either full or part time, with a schedule that may include weekends.

Education and Training

Dental assistants must have a high school diploma. Although many dental assistants learn their skills on the job, it has become more common for assistants to train in dental assisting programs at colleges, vocational schools, and technical institutes. These are one- or two-year programs that combine classroom lecture, laboratory experience, and preclinical instruction to help prepare students for work in a dental office. Graduates of programs accredited by the American Dental Association (ADA) can become licensed or registered dental assistants if they meet the requirements of their states.

In order to make yourself a more desirable candidate during a job search, consider becoming certified by an accredited organization via a certification exam. Two certification exams that are important for you to know about are the *certified dental assistant (CDA)* and the *registered dental assistant (RDA)*.

The ADA recognizes the Dental Assisting National Board (DANB) as the national certification and credentialing agency for dental assistants. DANB's national certificate and component exams meet regulatory requirements in 38 states. For those dental assistants who meet the eligibility and exam requirements, National DANB certification may be earned as a CDA. The CDA exam focuses on General Chairside Assisting and is DANB's primary certification. In addition to a General Chairside component, the CDA exam contains separate components covering Radiation Health and Safety and Infection Control topics. Many states are using the CDA exam or one of its components as part of dental assisting regulatory requirements. More than 100,000 certifications have been awarded and currently there are more than 30,000 professionals maintaining the credential.

The exam is offered in a computerized format throughout the year. DANB Exam Candidate Guides include information on how to apply for the exam(s), eligibility requirements, DANB policies, DANB exam applications, a listing of schools accredited by the Commission on Dental Accreditation (CODA), testing locations, a listing of DANB exam reference materials, and order forms for DANB study publications. Links to DANB Exam Candidate Guides can be found on the DANB website at www.danb.org.

An RDA is an educationally based, licensed credential. RDAs must graduate from an ADA-accredited dental assisting program, pass a comprehensive written and clinical exam, and maintain their license. The clinical portion of the RDA exam is supervised through the state dental board and is typically administered at a dental school. Some states will not recognize any outside testing agency, and in order to become an RDA, the dental assistant must take that state's RDA exam. Some of those states, however, do recognize DANB's standards for continuing education for RDAs.

Advancement Opportunities

With additional formal education or on-the-job training, a dental assistant can move up to become a Level II dental assistant or a dental hygienist, performing limited work on patients under the supervision of a dentist.

Without further education, advancement opportunities are limited. Some dental assistants who excel at working the front office become office managers.

For More Information

American Dental Assistants Association
35 E. Wacker Dr., Ste. 1730
Chicago, IL 60601-2211
(312) 541-1550
www.dentalassistant.org

American Dental Association
211 E. Chicago Ave.
Chicago, IL 60611-2678
(312) 440-2500
www.ada.org

National Association of Dental Assistants
900 S. Washington St., Ste. G13
Falls Church, VA 22046-4020
(703) 237-8616

MEDICAL ASSISTANT

Medical assisting is a challenging, rewarding profession. Medical assistants perform routine administrative and clinical tasks to keep hospitals, medical clinics, and the offices of physicians, podiatrists, chiropractors, dentists, optometrists, and other healthcare professionals running smoothly. Clinical and clerical duties vary from office to office depending on the office's size, location, and specialty. Medical assistants may perform any of the tasks listed below.

- ▶ While they may be restricted to typical office duties at a hospital, they may have clinical duties at a small clinic.
- ▶ Those who are strictly administrative may answer telephones, greet patients, update and file patient medical records, fill out insurance forms, schedule appointments, arrange for hospital admission and laboratory services, and handle billing and bookkeeping.
- ▶ Those who are strictly clinical may work with patients and do laboratory work. In most small offices, medical assistants may handle both types of work.
- ▶ Their clinical duties vary according to state law; these duties may include taking medical histories and recording vital signs, explaining treatment procedures to patients, preparing patients for examination, and assisting during routine examinations.
- ▶ They also collect and prepare laboratory specimens, perform basic lab tests, dispose of contaminated supplies, and sterilize medical instruments.
- ▶ They instruct patients about medication and special diets, prepare and administer medications, authorize drug refills, telephone prescriptions to a pharmacy, draw blood, prepare patients for x-rays, remove sutures, and change dressings.

▶ Some may take on the role of office manager, whose duties might include planning the doctor's schedule, taking dictation, overseeing a budget, and purchasing medical equipment.

As the healthcare industry continues to adjust to a growing patient population, more and more employers of allied health personnel insist that their medical assistants be certified as either a *certified medical assistant (CMA)* or a *registered medical assistant (RMA)*.

CMAs are certified through the American Association of Medical Assistants (AAMA). Becoming certified as a medical assistant increases your opportunities for career advancement, offers a professional edge, and confers greater prestige among coworkers and employers. To earn the official CMA credential you must enroll in a medical assisting program accredited by either the Commission on Accreditation of Allied Health Education Programs (CAAHEP) or the Accrediting Bureau of Health Education Schools (ABHES). During your schooling here, you will attain academic and clinical training in a variety of areas, including:

▶ human anatomy, physiology, and pathology
▶ medical terminology
▶ keyboarding and computer applications
▶ recordkeeping and accounting
▶ coding and insurance processing
▶ laboratory techniques
▶ clinical and diagnostic procedures
▶ pharmacology
▶ medication administration
▶ first aid
▶ office practices
▶ patient relations
▶ medical law and ethics

After graduating from the program, candidates must successfully complete the rigorous CMA Certification Examination. Achieving the credential demonstrates two important things to your employer. First, you possess exceptionally broad, thorough knowledge of the field in which you're working. Second, you care enough about your profession to attain that knowledge. The CMA credential must be renewed every five years, which means you have ongoing opportunities to learn about new developments in healthcare delivery.

In addition to having better job opportunities, CMAs typically receive higher wages and benefits. The CMA credential is a national certification recognized by employers across the country, so the time you invest in certification will pay off for you no matter where you end up. Find more information on the AAMA website at www.aama-ntl.org.

RMAs are awarded through the American Medical Technicians (AMT). To receive an RMA you must meet the prerequisite requirements, submit an application to take the RMA exam, and of course pass the exam. The prerequisites are:

1. You must be of good moral character.
2. You must meet one of the three following requirements:
   a. you must be a recent graduate from an accredited medical assistant program or a formal medical services training program of the United States Armed Forces;
   b. you must have been employed as a medical assistant for five years; or
   c. you must have passed a generalist medical assistant certification examination offered by another medical assisting certification body.

For more detailed information about the receiving RMA certification, visit AMT's website at www.amt1.com.

Typical Salaries

On average, medical assistants earn $22,000 to $29,000 or more annually working full time. Those with experience or an associate degree earn more than those without.

Typical Salaries for Medical Assistants in Different Areas

City	Low End	Average	High End
Charlotte, NC	23,704	28,516	32,833
El Paso, TX	20,987	25,018	29,070
Jacksonville, FL	22,775	26,729	31,547
Los Angeles, CA	26,947	31,691	37,325
Milwaukee, WI	25,268	29,529	34,999
New York, NY	28,463	33,905	39,425
San Francisco, CA	29,130	34,629	40,348

Source: www.swz.salary.com

Hiring Trends

Employment opportunities for medical assistants are projected to grow quickly through at least 2014. The aging U.S. population will place greater demand on the medical community, and the decreasing number of physicians means there will be a greater need for medical support staff, particularly those with formal training or experience.

Changes to medical billing codes and cost-cutting measures within the healthcare industry mean that more documentation will need to be done in less time and with fewer physicians. Physicians will increasingly rely on medical assistants to keep their practice running smoothly and to uphold high standards of patient care.

Most medical assistants work in the offices of physicians and other health practitioners such as chiropractors, optometrists, and podiatrists. Positions are available in hospitals, nursing homes, and other healthcare facilities.

Personal Abilities and Personality Traits Needed

Like all healthcare workers, medical assistants must have the desire to help people. They must be friendly, patient, and empathetic. Since medical assistants deal with the public, they must be neat and well groomed and have a courteous, pleasant manner. They must be able to put patients at ease, explain physicians' instructions, and respect the confidential nature of medical information. Confidentiality is a priority in the healthcare industry. Medical assistants have access to patient records and personal information, and must be able to maintain the highest standards of ethics.

A medical assistant's clinical duties require a reasonable level of manual dexterity as well as good eyesight. Medical assistants need to be computer-comfortable, as they may work with patients' electronic medical and health records, electronic prescriptions, databases, billing software, and electronic treatment protocols.

Doctors' offices, hospitals, and clinics are usually busy and fast paced. Medical assistants generally work 40 hours per week, including some evenings and weekends, and their work may vary greatly from day to day.

Education and Training

Medical assistants must have a high school diploma. Preference is given to candidates who have completed formal training; even so, much of the job training is completed on site. Many vocational schools and community colleges offer two-year programs leading to a medical assistant certificate or diploma.

As discussed earlier (see Description of Typical Duties), the AAMA and the AMT both offer registration into their organizations and professional certification to those assistants who meet training criteria and experience requirements and who pass a standardized test.

Advancement Opportunities

Medical assistants who have earned certification or who have more experience or training than their coworkers may advance into supervisory positions and assist with managing other medical assistants. Assistants may also move up to office management, administration, personnel management, or human resources management positions. Some assistants use their experience as a springboard into other healthcare careers such as nursing or medical technology.

For More Information

American Association of Medical Assistants
20 N. Wacker Dr., Ste. 1575
Chicago, IL 60606
(312) 899-1500
www.aama-ntl.org

American Medical Technicians
10700 W. Higgins Rd.
Rosemont, IL 60068
(847) 823-5169
www.amt1.com

NURSING ASSISTANT

Nursing assistants, also known as nursing aides or hospital attendants, work under the supervision of nursing and medical staff to complete patients' daily activities. Nursing homes, hospitals, adult day care centers, personal homes, and assisted living facilities all require nursing assistants to act as a helpful liaison between the RN (registered nurse) or LPN (licensed practical nurse) and the patient. In many cases, the nursing assistant serves as the RN's or LPN's eyes and ears. Nursing assistants perform indirect care and routine tasks.

► They work directly with patients—answering patient call bells, delivering messages, serving meals, making beds, and bathing and dressing, and assisting patients who need help to eat.

- ▶ They may also change patient dressings, apply lotion or ointment, and take patients' temperature, pulse, respiration, and blood pressure.
- ▶ They may also escort patients to operating and examining rooms, set up equipment, or store and move supplies.
- ▶ They may have to move patients in and out of bed or help them to stand or walk.

The nursing assistant works under supervision to provide basic needs for patients of any age, ethnicity, or gender. Since nursing assistants have daily contact with patients, they are key to providing vital information about the patients' condition to their supervisors. Nursing assistants may work in hospitals, nursing homes, long-term care facilities, clinics, and private residences. Those who work specifically with geriatric patients are called *geriatric nurse assistants.*

Home health aides (also known as *personal and home care aides*) provide medical treatment and personal care to patients in private home settings. Home health aides provide care and services that allow elderly, convalescent, or disabled persons to live in their own homes rather than in healthcare facilities. Under the direction of nursing or medical staff, they provide health-related services, such as administering oral medications. Like nursing aides, these aides may check patients' pulse rate, temperature, and respiration rate; help with simple prescribed exercises; and help patients to get in and out of bed, bathe, dress, and groom. Occasionally, they change nonsterile dressings, give massages and provide skin care, or assist with braces and artificial limbs. With training, experienced home health aides also may assist with medical equipment such as ventilators, which help patients breathe. Most home health aides work with elderly or disabled persons who need more extensive care than family or friends can provide. Some assist discharged hospital patients who have relatively short-term needs. In home health agencies, a registered nurse, physical therapist, or social worker usually assigns specific duties to and supervises home health aides, who keep records of the services they perform and record each patient's condition and progress. The aides report changes in a patient's condition to the supervisor or case manager.

Typical Salaries

On average, nursing assistants earn $23,000 to $29,000 or more annually working full time. Certified nursing assistants (CNAs) typically earn about $25,000 to $31,000.

Typical Salaries for Nursing Assistants in Different Areas

City	Low End	Average	High End
Charlotte, NC	20,443	26,033	32,330
El Paso, TX	18,100	22,393	28,625
Jacksonville, FL	19,642	25,131	31,064
Los Angeles, CA	23,240	29,184	36,753
Milwaukee, WI	21,792	27,553	34,463
New York, NY	24,548	31,657	38,821
San Francisco, CA	25,123	32,305	39,731

Source: www.swz.salary.com

Hiring Trends

The employment outlook for nursing aides and assistants is excellent, due in part to the increasing long-term care needs of an aging population. Additionally, nursing shortages in some healthcare systems mean more opportunities for assistants to supplement patient care and administration.

The United States is experiencing a nursing shortage that is expected to intensify as baby boomers age and the need for healthcare grows. A result of this problem is that nursing colleges and universities across the country are struggling to expand enrollment levels to meet the rising demand for nursing care. The U.S. nursing shortage is projected to grow to over 250,000 registered nurses by 2025.

As the average age of the registered nurse increases, the size of the nursing workforce is expected to plateau when large numbers of RNs retire. Demand for RNs is expected to increase during this time, resulting in a large and prolonged shortage of nurses that is expected to affect the U.S. healthcare industry even further within the next decade.

Patients will continue to need healthcare services regardless of the nursing shortage; this will open more professional opportunities for nursing assistants and nursing aides well into the next decade.

Personal Abilities and Personality Traits Needed

Nursing assistants often have more contact with patients than other members of the healthcare team, so it is important that they be tactful, patient, understanding, emotionally stable, and dependable. And, as stated previously, they should of course have a desire to help people. Assistants should also be able to work as part of a team and be willing to perform repetitive, routine tasks.

They need to be strong enough to assist with supporting patients during transfer from bed to chair or wheelchair, with no serious back or shoulder problems that would limit their ability to carry out patient support tasks.

Additionally, nursing assistants who work as home health aides must have reliable transportation, be able to work independently, keep accurate records, and have excellent time management skills. Home health aides may be supervised by a registered nurse, a nurse manager, or sometimes a physician.

Education and Training

Nursing assistants must have a high school diploma or a GED (General Education Development) certificate and, in some states or healthcare systems, CNA certification. Certification is earned by completing a 6-to-12-week program at a community college, vocational school, or medical facility. Students study basic nursing principles and skills, anatomy and physiology, nutrition, infection control, computer skills, and laboratory operations; they also experience hands-on clinical activities.

Although certification is not required in all locations, assistants who are certified have a competitive edge over noncertified applicants. A certificate is given for completion of a training program that focuses on a particular technical skill or job. Such programs usually last from six months to one year and can be taken after high school. You can receive certificate training in an educational setting—such as a community college, technical school or university—or in a job setting, such as a hospital or a health clinic.

The CNA title carries a high level of experience and ability; however, issues of liability and legality prevent the CNA from performing certain procedures. Most training for the CNA is accomplished through programs offered by the Red Cross, community colleges, and online schools and through medical facilities. The latter option provides on-the-job training that is valuable for any nursing assistant. Many schools offer training within medical facilities as part of their course programs as well. All CNAs must take an examination before they become qualified nursing assistants.

Nursing shortages offer the nursing assistant many challenges. The job can have a high level of stress, and turnover rates for the profession are high because of this shortage. On the other hand, this shortage provides more jobs for those who are intent on working in this job. The demand for CNAs is high, especially among those institutions that provide quality care to the elderly. Many healthcare facilities recognize the important role that a qualified CNA can play in the quality of care they offer. Additionally, a CNA can find support through organizations such as the National Association of Health Care Assistants.

The important thing to remember is that states differ with regard to the amount of time required for training and testing and the environment in which you would be working. Before you begin your nursing assistant training, contact your State Nurse Aide Registry and/or State Licensing Board to learn about their requirements. You also might check to make sure you meet the requirements for nursing assistants in any state where you would like to work.

Advancement Opportunities

For nursing aides, opportunities for advancement are limited. To enter other health occupations, aides generally need additional formal training. Some employers and unions provide opportunities by simplifying the educational paths to advancement. Experience as an aide can also help you decide whether to pursue additional training for another career in the healthcare field.

For More Information

American Association of Colleges of Nursing
One Dupont Circle, NW, Ste. 530
Washington, DC 20036
(202) 463-6930
www.aacn.nche.edu

The National Association for Home Care and Hospice
228 Seventh St., SE
Washington, DC 20003
(202) 547-7424
www.nahc.org/

Nursing Aide Assistant Guides
www.nursingassistantguides.com

PHYSICAL THERAPY ASSISTANT

Physical therapy assistants (PTAs), also known as physical therapy aides, work under the supervision of physical therapists (PTs) to prepare patients both physically and psychologically for therapy, and instruct patients in a wide variety of treatments. They use physical therapy techniques to help improve mobility, strength, and flexibility; relieve pain; and restore functioning after disease, injury, or trauma. They work in hospitals, nursing homes, long-term care facilities, rehabilitation clinics, or medical clinics. They are members of a healthcare team that may include doctors, occupational therapists, speech therapists, neurologists, social workers, and recreation therapists.

Physical therapist assistants work with people of all ages, from children to the elderly. They may specialize by patient population (such as geriatrics or pediatrics), treatment modality (such as massage or exercise), patient condition (such as post stroke, arthritis, or amputation), or they may work with all types of patients.

Specific duties may include any of the following.

▶ They may aid patients who need to exercise on a treadmill or stationary bike or in a swimming pool or use weight-lifting equipment.
▶ They help administer massages, electrical stimulation, paraffin baths, hot/cold packs, and traction.
▶ They may measure a patient's size, flexibility, and range of motion or use ultrasound equipment to evaluate patients' discomfort in a knee, elbow, or other joint.
▶ Most importantly, they encourage patients during therapy sessions and make sure they perform exercises correctly to achieve maximum benefit and avoid further injury.

In addition to providing therapy, assistants educate patients on the proper care and use of assistive equipment and devices, such as lifts, walkers, wheelchairs, and artificial limbs.

Typical Salaries

On average, licensed physical therapy assistants earn $32,000 to $46,000 or more annually working full time, depending on their years of experience. Nonlicensed physical therapy aides make considerably less.

Typical Salaries for Licensed Physical Therapy Assistants in Different Areas

City	Low End	Average	High End
Charlotte, NC	34,383	42,115	51,078
El Paso, TX	30,442	37,076	45,307
Jacksonville, FL	33,036	40, 980	49, 167
Los Angeles, CA	39,087	48,753	58,173
Milwaukee, WI	36,652	45,395	54,549
New York, NY	41,286	51,215	61,446
San Francisco, CA	42,254	52,298	62,886

Source: www.swz.salary.com

Hiring Trends

As with other types of healthcare assistant careers, opportunities for physical therapist assistants are expected to grow rapidly at least through 2014. This growth will be fueled by an aging population that will require more physical therapy for a longer period of time and a shortage of physical therapists in many areas, which makes licensed assistants an attractive alternative.

More than half of all assistants and aides work in hospitals or private physical therapy offices. Others work in clinics, nursing homes, and even inside patients' homes. In sports medicine, they may work part time on the sidelines or in swimming pools performing aquatherapy.

Personal Abilities and Personality Traits Needed

Physical therapy is almost always conducted in a clean, energizing environment. Physical therapist assistants need to be neat, professional, upbeat, and patient.

Some patients are depressed or angry about their need for treatment, and an important part of the assistant's job is being able to offer encouragement and enthusiasm for small successes.

Assistants need a moderate amount of physical strength and stamina to assist patients with treatment. Constant kneeling, stooping, and standing are all part of the job. In some cases, assistants may need to help lift patients, so those prone to back problems are strongly advised not to become physical therapy assistants.

Most physical therapist assistants work 40 hours per week, some on the weekends.

As physical therapy evolves, therapeutic equipment and devices will become more electronic and technologically advanced. Therapist assistants need to have at least basic computer skills in order to keep up with changing technology.

Education and Training

Physical therapist assistants must have a high school degree. In many cases an associate degree is required. Courses in mathematics, fitness theory, anatomy, and science will help prepare a candidate for work as an assistant.

Qualifications for licensure vary from state to state, but all require that a candidate have earned at least a high school diploma and some hands-on, supervised experience in a clinical setting. Some states require physical therapy assistants to be licensed before they can practice; others do not require it but many employers expect it. Many individuals who seek to gain a physical therapy assistant license also elect to enroll in accredited associate degree programs in physical therapy. These programs typically consist of four semesters and include both classroom instruction on medical basics (such as biology, anatomy, and chemistry) as well as clinical experience. Some states also require that candidates seeking a PTA license complete basic certification in CPR and first aid. These courses can be offered either as part of an associate degree or individually through community centers and vocational schools.

The Federation of State Boards of Physical Therapy (FSBPT) develops and administers the National Physical Therapy Examination (NPTE) for both physical therapists and physical therapy assistants in 53 jurisdictions—all 50 states, the District of Columbia, Puerto Rico, and the Virgin Islands. These high-stakes exams assess the basic entry-level competence for first-time licensure or registration as a PT or PTA. Candidates interested in licensure can register for an exam, download a candidate handbook, authorize release of exam scores, and complete other functions related to licensure on the FSBPT website at www.fsbpt.org.

Advancement Opportunities

With specific training, physical therapy aides can advance to licensed physical therapist assistants; with more training, they can eventually can become physical therapists. Licensed physical therapy assistants can administer many more aspects of the treatment prescribed by the therapist than can unlicensed aides.

For More Information

American Physical Therapy Association
1111 N Fairfax St.
Alexandria, VA 22314-1488
(800) 999-2782
www.apta.org

Federation of State Boards of Physical Therapy
509 Wythe St.
Alexandria, VA 22314
(703) 299-3100
www.fsbpt.org

National Rehabilitation Association
633 S Washington St.
Alexandria, VA 22314-4109
(703) 836-0850
www.nationalrehab.org

RADIOLOGIC TECHNICIAN

There are three different types of radiologic technicians: radiographers, radiation therapy technicians, and sonographers.

Radiographers
▶ Radiographers produce x-ray films of parts of the human body for use in diagnosing medical problems.
▶ They prepare patients for radiologic exams by explaining the procedure, removing any jewelry, and positioning patients so the correct body part can be radiographed.
▶ They place the x-ray film under the part of the patient's body to be examined and make the exposure.
▶ They then remove the film and develop it.

Radiation Therapy Technicians
▶ Radiation therapy technnicians prepare cancer patients for treatment and administer prescribed doses of ionizing radiation to specific body parts.
▶ They position patients under high-energy linear accelerators to expose affected body parts to treatment.
▶ They check the patient for radiation side effects such as nausea, hair loss, and skin irritation.
▶ They give instructions and explanations to patients who are likely to be very ill.

Sonographers
▶ Sonographers, also known as ultrasound technicians, use machines that project high-frequency sound waves into areas of the patient's body that reflect echoes and form an image.
▶ They explain the procedure to the patient, record additional medical history, and position the patient for testing.
▶ They look for subtle differences between healthy and pathological areas.

Typical Salaries

On average, radiologic technicians earn $37,000 to $53,000 or more annually, working full time, depending on their education level and length of training.

Typical Salaries for Radiologic Technicians in Different Areas

City	Low End	Average	High End
Charlotte, NC	38,684	46,368	54,635
El Paso, TX	34,251	41,512	48,373
Jacksonville, FL	37,169	44,708	52,495
Los Angeles, CA	43,977	50,655	62,110
Milwaukee, WI	41,237	49,163	58,240
New York, NY	46,451	55,874	65,604
San Francisco, CA	47,540	57,066	67,142

Source: www.swz.salary.com

Hiring Trends

Employment of radiologic technicians is expected to grow well beyond 2012. Current and new uses of imaging equipment will increase demand. Radiologic technicians are chiefly employed by hospitals.

Personal Abilities and Personality Traits Needed

Technicians are on their feet for long periods and may lift or turn disabled patients frequently. They work at machines but may also do some procedures at patients' bedsides. They must follow precise physician instructions and regulations concerning use of radiation to ensure that they themselves, patients, and coworkers are protected from overexposure.

Even more so than other radiologic technicians radiation therapists must be patient and sensitive. They may be more prone to emotional burnout because they regularly treat extremely ill and dying patients.

Education and Training

Depending on your background and goals, you may enter the radiation technology career with a certificate, an associate degree, or a bachelor's degree. Since many states mandate licensure for radiation technicians, be sure to verify that the radiation therapy program you are considering is accredited. Many radiation technicians earn an associate or bachelor's degree in radiology and then earn a 12-month certificate in radiation therapy. Radiation therapy programs include training in radiation therapy procedures and the science that underlies them. Examples of course topics include anatomy, physiology, physics, precalculus, writing, and research methods. State licensing for radiation technicians often requires the candidate to pass a certification exam through the American Registry of Radiologic Technicians (ARRT).

In accordance with ARRT's *Equation for Excellence*, candidates for ARRT certification must meet basic requirements in the three components: ethics, education, and examination.

> **Ethics**—According to the governing documents shown on the ARRT website (www.arrt.org) every candidate for certification and every applicant for renewal of registration must "be a person of good moral character and must not have engaged in conduct that is inconsistent with the ARRT Rules of Ethics," and must "agree to comply with the ARRT Rules and Regulations and the ARRT Standards of Ethics." ARRT investigates all potential violations in order to determine eligibility. Further information may be found on the ARRT website and in the handbooks for each discipline, which are available on the site.
> **Education**—Candidates for certification must satisfactorily complete certain formal educational requirements by an accredited body and must demonstrate competency in coursework and an ARRT-specified list of

clinical procedures. Further details may be found in the handbooks for each of the post-primary certification disciplines; these handbooks are available on the ARRT website.

Examination—The final step in the certification process is to pass an examination developed and administered by the ARRT. The exams assess the knowledge and cognitive skills underlying the intelligent perform-ance of the tasks typically required of staff technicians practicing within the respective disciplines. Exam content is specified on the ARRT web-site and in the respective handbook for each discipline.

Advancement Opportunities

With experience and additional training, staff technicians may become spe-cialists and may be promoted to supervisor, chief radiologic technician, or department administrator or director. Some technicians progress by becom-ing instructors or directors in radiologic technology programs; others take jobs as sales representatives or instructors with equipment manufacturers.

Radiation therapy technicians can specialize as medical radiation *dosimetrists*. A medical dosimetrist is a member of the radiation oncology team who has knowledge of the overall of radiation oncology treatment ma-chines and equipment, is knowledgeable about common procedures, and has the education and expertise necessary to develop treatment plans in col-laboration with radiation oncologists.

Sonographers advance by specializing in a particular area: neurosonogra-phy (the brain and nervous system), vascular (blood flow), echocardiography (the heart), abdominal (the liver, kidneys, spleen, and pancreas), obstetrics/gynecology (the female reproductive system), or ophthalmosonography (the eye). Abdominal sonographers use sonography to inspect patients' ab-domens. They look for abnormalities or disease in the liver, pancreas, kid-neys, spleen, gallbladder, and bile ducts, and also use the technology as a means of treatment, determining whether the current course of therapy has been effective. In some cases they may scan parts of the chest as well, but this area is usually left to the echocardiographer.

Neurosonagraphers specialize in the areas of the brain and the nervous sys-tem. They diagnose disorders of the nervous system and abnormalities in the brain, such as tumors. They may also scan for evidence of strokes. Neurosonographers use a slightly different technology than obstetric or abdominal sonographers to produce their scans.

Ophthalmic sonographers study the eyes. They diagnose tumors, detached retinas, and other diseases of the eye. They can also provide accurate measurements of the eye for the insertion of prosthetics. The technology used in ophthalmic sonography is specific to the practice; it is much smaller than that used by other areas.

Echocardiographers deal specifically with the heart. They use ultrasound technology to get an accurate picture of the heart, which can be done while the patient is resting or active. These pictures, called *echocardiograms*, are used to examine the chambers, valves, and vessels of the heart and to identify any abnormalities or disorders.

Vascular technicians deal with similar areas, mainly the circulatory system. They use the ultrasound technology to check blood flow and circulation, blood pressure, and oxygen saturation. These tests are usually run during or immediately after surgery to ensure that every organ is getting the amount of blood it needs to function properly, and also to check for any abnormalities in the amount of blood flowing to certain areas.

In addition to performing the scans, sonographers are also responsible for keeping accurate patient records and being able to analyze the information obtained in the scans for diagnosis and treatment. They also maintain their own equipment, and may be responsible for the purchase of new equipment, as well as keeping abreast of any technological advances. Some sonographers may become department supervisors, responsible for the actions and operation of the entire sonography team.

Sonography is a growing opportunity in the medical field, expected to increase more quickly than any other area, especially as technology and uses expand. It can also lead to several opportunities outside the hospital or private practice, including research and education. Not limited to the practice of obstetrics, it can be an exciting and rewarding profession, both professionally and personally.

Five Steps to Becoming an Ultrasound Specialist

Step One: Earn a high school diploma. Ultrasound, or sonography, training programs require that applicants have earned a high school diploma or its equivalent. Good courses to prepare for ultrasound specialist training include biology, anatomy, physics, advanced math, and computer science.

Step Two: Complete an ultrasound training program. CAAHEP (www.caahep.org) has accredited approximately 150 training programs for ultrasound specialists. The majority are associate degree programs that include coursework in physiology, anatomy, simple physics, equipment operation, and patient care.

Step Three: Become certified. Although licensure isn't always required to work as an ultrasound specialist, most employers prefer to hire job candidates who are certified and registered.

Step Four: Develop a specialization. Ultrasound technicians advance by developing expertise in specialized areas, such as obstetric and gynecological sonography or abdominal sonography. A candidate demonstrates specialist credentials to employers by becoming registered in the specialty through the American Registry for Diagnostic Medical Sonography (ARDMS).

Step Five: Broaden your skills. Many ultrasound specialists pursue multiple specializations to enhance their marketability. Research, sales, and education are other fields in which ultrasound specialists can advance their careers.

SURGICAL TECHNICIAN

Surgical technicians, also called surgical or operating room technicians, assist in operations under the supervision of surgeons, registered nurses, or other surgical personnel.

- ▶ Before an operation, surgical technicians help set up the operating room with surgical instruments and equipment, sterile linens, and sterile solutions.
- ▶ They assemble, adjust, and check nonsterile equipment to ensure that it is working properly.
- ▶ They prepare patients for surgery by washing, shaving, and disinfecting incision sites on patients.
- ▶ They transport patients to the operating room, help position them on the operating table, and cover them with sterile surgical drapes.

▶ They observe patients' vital signs, check charts, and help the surgical team scrub and put on gloves, gowns, and masks.

Essentially, a surgical technician's main goal is to help surgical procedures run smoothly. Technicians work with a team of physicians, nurses, surgeons, and anesthesiologists in order to ensure a smooth procedure. Surgical tech jobs can be found within most hospitals, though some private facilities may also employ technicians. In addition, physicians may employ technicians if they require additional assistance.

Surgical tech jobs are very demanding physically and emotionally, since operating rooms tend to be high-stress areas. In addition to wearing surgical scrubs at all times, technicians must also be on their feet for the better part of a work day. Most universities do not offer specific surgical technician programs, though some technical schools offer classes that can be applied toward surgical tech jobs. A college, technical, or university degree is not required in order to secure a surgical tech job, though the vast majority of surgical technicians have obtained a high school diploma or an associate degree. Additional on-site training may be offered at some hospital locations. All surgical technicians should have basic math skills in addition to some surgical or medical knowledge.

The National Board of Surgical Technology and Surgical Assisting (NBSTSA) was established in 1974 as the certifying agency for Surgical technicians. NBSTSA is solely responsible for all decisions regarding certification, from determining eligibility to maintaining, denying, granting, and renewing the designation. Certification as a surgical technician or a first assistant demonstrates that an individual meets the national standard for knowledge set forth by the organization. Certification, which is often a requirement for employment, can lead to advancement in the profession as well as to higher pay.

To be eligible for the certification exam, candidates must provide either evidence of current or previous certification as a surgical technician or documentation of graduation from a surgical technology program accredited by either CAAHEP or ABHES. For a list of CAAHEP-approved surgical technology programs go to www.caahep.org; for a list of ABHES-approved surgical technology programs go to www.abhes.org.

Before testing, individuals must establish eligibility by submitting the appropriate application form along with the required fees. Once eligibility to test has been established, approved candidates will be provided with information with which to contact the testing agency to schedule the date, time, and location for testing.

Typical Salaries

On average, surgical technicians earn between $28,000 and $40,000 or more annually, working full time, depending on their training and experience.

Typical Salaries for Surgical Technicians in Different Areas

City	Low End	Average	High End
Charlotte, NC	32,074	39,497	47,075
El Paso, TX	28,398	35,381	41,680
Jacksonville, FL	30,817	37,106	45,231
Los Angeles, CA	36,462	45,280	53,515
Milwaukee, WI	34,190	40,839	50,181
New York, NY	38,513	47,624	56,526
San Francisco, CA	39,416	48,622	57,851

Source: www.swz.salary.com

Hiring Trends

As the volume of surgery increases and operating room staffing patterns change, employment for surgical technicians is expected to increase until at least 2012.

Most surgical technicians are employed by hospitals, mainly in operating and delivery rooms. Some, called private scrubs, are employed directly by surgeons who have special surgical teams.

Technological advances will continue to require more surgical procedures, and the movement to outpatient or ambulatory surgery will mean rapid growth in demand for surgical technicians in physicians' offices and clinics, including surgical centers.

Personal Abilities and Personality Traits Needed

Surgical technicians work in clean, well-lighted, and cool environments. They must stand for long periods of time. At times they may be exposed to communicable diseases and unpleasant sights, odors, and materials.

Surgical technicians need manual dexterity to handle instruments quickly.

They must also be conscientious, orderly, and emotionally stable in order to handle the demands of the operating room environment.

Surgical technicians must respond quickly and know procedures well, so they can get instruments ready for surgeons without having to be told.

Advancement Opportunities

Surgical technicians advance by specializing in a particular area of surgery, such as neurosurgery or open heart surgery. Specialization is acquired through on-the-job training in a clinical setting.

They may also work as circulating technicians or nonsterile members of surgical teams, preparing patients, helping with anesthesia, obtaining, opening, and holding packages for the sterile workers during procedures, interviewing patients before surgery, and so on. With additional training, some technicians advance to become first assistants, who help with retracting, sponging, suturing, cauterizing bleeders, and closing and treating wounds; others become RNs.

For More Information

National Board of Surgical Technology and Surgical Assisting
6 W. Dry Creek Cir., Ste. 100
Littleton, CO 80120
(800) 707-0057
www.nbstsa.org

HOW TO BECOME A HEALTHCARE WORKER

The healthcare field is an explosive arena for job growth. Many hospitals and other doctors' practices are continually seeking to fill entry-level positions such as dental assistant, medical assistant, nursing assistant, physical therapy assistant, surgical technician, and radiologic technician are the positions.

You can enter and succeed in these occupations by following these steps:

- ▶ Graduate from high school or obtain a GED.
- ▶ Conduct a self-evaluation.
- ▶ Decide on an area of specialization.
- ▶ Find a training program that suits your needs.
- ▶ Complete the training program.
- ▶ Conduct your job search.
- ▶ Succeed in your first job.
- ▶ Make professional connections whenever you can.
- ▶ Find a mentor.
- ▶ Specialize.
- ▶ Pursue advanced certification or license.

In almost every city, the local public school system offers youth apprenticeships that guide high school students into the healthcare field with firsthand experience and a certificate that helps them get a job or enter a training program immediately after graduation. You may also be able to find an internship or volunteer opportunities by contacting hospitals, clinics, and private medical practices in your area. Approach your search with the same seriousness and professionalism you would a job search. Ask whom to speak with regarding internship/volunteer opportunities and be prepared to discuss your interest, your qualifications, and your career goals, as well as provide personal and employment references.

If you are not in a high school or apprenticeship program, the first step to becoming a healthcare worker is to graduate from high school or earn a GED, which you can do through any adult education center in your area.

Since there are many areas of specialization in the healthcare field, you need to decide where you might fit in best. Writing a self-evaluation will help you pinpoint your abilities and personality traits.

Evaluating Yourself

Your self-evaluation will help show you a path to take. Your strengths and weaknesses can guide you, so take this step seriously and devote as much time to it as you need. Begin your evaluation by deciding how much training you wish to pursue and commit to. (See Chapter 2 for detailed information on all these types of programs.)

Also, think about your areas of interest and what you do well. What skills do you most enjoy using? Write down your skills, gifts, and talents, and then prioritize them. List all the jobs you have ever had, including summer jobs, volunteer work, part-time jobs, and any freelance or short-term assignments. Then add a similar list of your hobbies and other activities, including any special experiences you have had, such as babysitting or travel.

Do the same for your education, listing the school(s) you attended, your major courses of study, grades, special awards or honors, courses you particularly enjoyed, and extracurricular activities. These lists may begin to show you a likely career pattern.

Work environment is another key consideration in choosing a healthcare career. Consider whether you prefer to work in a subset of a large, busy organization or a small office practice. Do you prefer a city, suburb, or a rural location? What part of the country do you want to stay in or move to?

An experienced counselor can be of great help in the decision-making process. Counselors can give you a series of vocational interest and aptitude tests, and can interpret and explain the results. Vocational testing and counseling are offered in guidance departments of high schools, vocational schools, and colleges. Some local offices of the state employment services affiliated with the federal employment service offer free counseling. Counselors will not tell you what to do, but they can help guide you in your search for a specialization.

Evaluating yourself will help tell you what type of job you are likely to excel in. You also may find it helpful to keep in mind your answers to the following questions:

▶ Do you want to work with patients or with machines?
▶ Do you prefer to work on a team or individually?
▶ Do you want good benefits or a chance for quick promotion?
▶ Do you want a variety of tasks or a few routine duties?
▶ What is the level of your physical stamina or strength?

Compare your answers with the descriptions of jobs listed earlier in this chapter to find a match.

Types of Employers

For each healthcare position discussed in this book, there are many different types of employers. The most general employer is a hospital, offering a multitude of positions for entry-level job seekers.

Hospitals are described as short-stay or long-term, depending on how much time a patient spends there before being discharged.

▶ The most common type of hospital is the *community* or *general hospital*, typically a small hospital where most people receive care.
▶ A *teaching hospital* provides clinical training for medical students and other medical professionals and is usually part of a major medical school.
▶ *Public hospitals* are owned and operated by federal, state, or city governments, are usually located in the inner cities, and often treat patients who are unable to pay for services or who depend on Medicaid payments.

In *group medical practices*, which are very common, two or more doctors share a building or office, but each doctor may have a separate staff. The doctors share the expenses of the building. Group practices may include optometrists, chiropractors, dentists, or other professionals and can range from large organizations to small offices with one or two assistants.

Health maintenance organizations (HMOs) are group practices organized to provide complete coverage for subscribers' health needs at a pre-established price. The patients (or their employers) pay a set amount each month; in turn, the HMO group provides care such as routine checkups at no extra charge, or at a very minimal charge. Members are usually locked into the plan for a specified period of time—usually one year—and if the service they need is available within the HMO, they must use a selected HMO doctor.

Mental health facilities provide medication, emotional support, and physical support to mentally ill patients.

Hospices provide support and care for terminally ill people in the final stage of their disease so they can live as comfortably and fully as possible. A hospice offers a program of services for both patients and their families so they can make the necessary preparations for death. A hospice may be a freestanding institution, a special wing at a hospital, or simply a few beds that can be made available to the program as needed.

Home healthcare provides nursing services in patients' homes. Patients may be any age and include those who expect to get better and resume work and daily activities as well as those who expect to die. Care may include everything from giving medication to providing physical therapy to housekeeping.

Nursing homes provide long-term care for elderly patients. There are three types of nursing homes.

▶ A *residential care facility* normally provides meals and housekeeping for the resident, plus some basic medical monitoring, and is geared toward residents who are fairly independent and do not need constant medical attention.

▶ An *intermediate care facility* offers room and board and nursing care as necessary for those who can no longer live independently.

A skilled nursing facility provides round-the-clock nursing care plus physician coverage and is for patients who need intensive care plus services such as occupational therapy, physical therapy, and rehabilitation.

Each of these facilities provides exercise and social programs as well.

Surgicenters, also called *outpatient centers*, are ambulatory surgery centers equipped to perform routine surgical procedures that do not require an overnight stay. A surgicenter does not need the sophisticated and expensive equipment found in a hospital operating room. Minor surgery, such as abortions, tissue biopsies, hernia repair, cataract surgery, and some forms of cosmetic surgery are typically performed in these facilities.

Emergency clinics, also known as *urgent care clinics* are usually run by private for-profit organizations and provide up to 24-hour care on a drop-in basis. They offer quick help in an emergency when the nearest hospital is miles away, and they are usually open during the hours that most doctors' offices are closed. To minimize costs, they do not provide hospital beds. They deal with problems such as cuts that require sutures, sprains and bruises from accidents, and various infections.

OTHER HEALTHCARE JOB DESCRIPTIONS

The following job descriptions will give you an idea of what is involved in many healthcare fields. You can become an aide or an assistant in any of these specialty positions. Instead of a physical therapy assistant, you could become an art therapy assistant if arts and sciences are your strengths, or you could work as an assistant in the private practice of a dance therapist. You could become a medical assistant employed by an audiologist, a genetics counselor, or a chiropractor. You could become a surgical technician in a hospital or for an emergency clinic. The industry offers numerous possibilities. If you feel that healthcare is the field for you, read on to explore the many different avenues you can take to explore your passion.

► *Art therapists* are trained in the fine arts and the behavioral sciences to develop rehabilitation programs that use art materials and a variety of techniques such as painting, sculpting with clay, or making crafts.

▶ *Audiologists* test, diagnose, and treat people who have hearing and related problems.

▶ *Biochemists* study and research the chemical composition of living things, focusing on processes such as metabolism, reproduction, growth, and heredity.

▶ *Biomedical engineers* use engineering skills and concepts to invent or improve devices, instruments, and substances (such as pacemakers, ultrasound, or artificial limbs) used in treating medical problems.

▶ *Blood bank technicians* are medical technicians who specialize in the skills and knowledge needed to maintain a blood bank, such as drawing, classifying, testing, analyzing, and storing blood.

▶ *Cardiopulmonary technicians* conduct tests and evaluations related to the diagnosis and treatment of heart (cardiac) and lung (pulmonary) diseases and disorders.

▶ *Cardiovascular technicians* assist physicians and other medical personnel in diagnosing and treating medical problems related to the body's heart (cardiac) and blood vessel (peripheral vascular) systems.

▶ *Chiropractors* diagnose and treat medical problems related to the body's muscular, nervous, and skeletal systems, especially the spine.

▶ *Dance therapists* are trained in dance/movement, psychology, and physiology to treat and rehabilitate patients with emotional or physical disorders or developmental disabilities.

▶ *Dental hygienists* perform preventive dental procedures, including cleaning teeth, and instruct patients on oral hygiene practices to prevent teeth and gum abnormalities or disease.

▶ *Dentists* diagnose, prevent, and treat problems of the teeth and tissues of the mouth.

▶ *Dietitians* plan nutrition programs and supervise meal preparation and service, often for large institutions such as hospitals, schools, nursing homes, and prisons.

▶ *EEG technicians* conduct tests using EEG (electroencephalograph) equipment, which records electrical impulses in the brain, to assist neurologists (physicians who study the brain) in treating patients with neural disorders such as brain tumors, strokes, and Alzheimer's disease.

▶ *EKG technicians* are cardiovascular technicians who perform EKG (electrocardiogram) testing to record and monitor electrical impulses transmitted by the heart.

▶ *Genetic counselors* advise patients, often prospective parents, on matters related to hereditary diseases and disorders such as Down's syndrome, muscular dystrophy, and prebirth spinal or organ malformations.

▶ *Licensed practical nurses* provide basic nursing care (both medical and nonmedical) to sick, injured, convalescing, and handicapped patients under the direction of physicians and registered nurses.

▶ *Medical illustrators* use artistic skills and medical and anatomical knowledge to create drawings, diagrams, models, and other graphic aids for use in medical research, publications, consultations, exhibits, teaching, and various communications media.

▶ *Optometrists* diagnose and treat vision problems, prescribing and fitting eyeglasses and contact lenses, and may provide basic care for eye disorders such as cataracts and glaucoma (unlike ophthalmologists, who are physicians specializing in the treatment of eye diseases and injuries).

▶ *Orthotists* design, build, and fit devices to support weak body parts or correct physical defects, such as limb or spinal cord disorders stemming from cerebral palsy, polio, or stroke.

▶ *Pharmacists* dispense drugs prescribed by physicians and other medical practitioners, advise patients about medications, and consult with physicians about the selection, dosages, and effects of medications.

▶ *Physical therapists* rehabilitate people who suffer from physical disabilities caused by accidents or disease, using massage, water instruction, machine movement, or other methods.

▶ *Podiatrists* are doctors who diagnose and treat disorders, diseases, and injuries of the foot and lower leg.

▶ *Prosthetists* design, build, and fit artificial limbs (prostheses) for patients who have lost part or all of their own limbs through accident, illness, or a congenital condition.

▶ *Psychologists* study human behavior and mental processes to understand, explain, and change people's behavior, often within an area of specialty such as clinical, developmental, organizational, or research psychology.

▶ *Recreation therapists* use games, sports, exercises, arts and crafts, and other recreational activities to treat patients with emotional, physical, or mental disorders and help them develop effective social and interpersonal skills.

▶ *Registered nurses* provide direct and indirect patient care, including assessing, planning, implementing, and evaluating care in areas ranging from pediatrics to geriatrics.

▶ *Respiratory therapists* evaluate, treat, and care for patients with breathing disorders such as asthma and emphysema and provide emergency care for heart failure, stroke, drowning, or shock victims.

TYPICAL HIRING PROCEDURES

Among most hospitals and physicians' centers, the hiring procedures are about the same. Applicants normally fill out an application for employment and participate in an interview. Many employers prefer that applicants fill out the application on site, so remember to bring all necessary information you may not readily recall. You should also bring along several copies of your resume, and submit one with your application. The human resources representative or employment recruiter may talk briefly with you when you turn in your application. Bringing everything with you will impress the employment recruiter—it shows you are responsible, prepared, and have put thought into your interview.

For most positions, employers will request that you take a drug test and a physical. Also, they will usually conduct a criminal background check and screen your references.

At certain hospitals and other institutions, you cannot apply for a position unless it has been posted on the job board or applications have been requested in some other way. You may be offered a job description that outlines the duties and experience required for the position. Job titles may vary at different institutions, but the duties involved will be similar.

Here is a sample job posting for a medical assistant at a hospital.

MEDICAL ASSISTANT
(OR PATIENT CARE TECHNICIAN)

JOB SUMMARY:

Provides direct patient care under the direction of a registered nurse or licensed practical nurse according to policy and procedure. Contributes to the safe and effective operation of the nursing unit. Provides direct patient care primarily for patients ages 12 and up.

EDUCATION:

High school diploma or equivalent

LICENSURE:

None

EXPERIENCE:

Previous exposure to training

SKILLS:

Skills basic to completion of medical assistant course

ESSENTIAL PHYSICAL AND MENTAL FUNCTIONS AND
ENVIRONMENTAL CONDITIONS:

Able to see objects closely, as in reading, frequently. Able to see objects far away frequently. Able to discriminate color and perceive depth frequently. Able to hear normal sounds with some background noise, as in answering telephone, frequently. Able to distinguish sounds, as in voice patterns, frequently. Able to give and receive verbal communications continuously. Able to read and write written communications continuously. Able to carry objects weighing 10 pounds or more frequently; able to carry objects weighing 49 pounds or less on occasion. Able to sit 30 minutes consecutively, 1 hour per shift. Able to stand in place 10 minutes consecutively, 1 hour per shift. Able to remain on feet 4 hours consecutively, 7 hours per shift. Able to sustain awkward position 5 minutes consecutively, 2 hours per shift. Able to perform motor skills such as bending, twisting, turning, kneeling, reaching out, reaching up, wrist turning, grasping, finger manipulation, feeling perception, fast response, frequently.

Job openings are posted at hospitals for about five days, on average, and may be updated weekly. Many hospitals offer a job hotline number so prospective employees can keep up with the job openings. Smaller practices may take out ads in the newspapers or consult local hospitals for applicants.

The Application

The application for an entry-level position in healthcare is similar to an application for any kind of job, school, or financial aid.

The application will ask for the following information:

- ▶ name, address, and social security number
- ▶ job information or previous work experience, including dates and reason for leaving
- ▶ skills or supervisory experience
- ▶ educational experience
- ▶ references (or you may be asked to sign a references release statement)
- ▶ citizenship status

No question on the application should touch on a prospective employee's race, color, religion, national origin, age, sex, marital status, or disabilities. If there is such a question, you may leave it blank. The application should state that the company is an equal opportunity employer.

You will be asked to sign the application to verify that all the information is true and correct. The application will state that incorrect information is cause for immediate dismissal. Remember that the employer will verify the information, so it is best to be honest.

Your application will stay active on file at a hospital for six months. In smaller healthcare practices, your application may or may not remain on file, depending on the size of the practice. Smaller practices usually do not have as high a turnover rate as hospitals, so there is little need to keep applications on file.

Employment Agencies

Employment agencies use the same hiring techniques as other companies. You will fill out an application, the agency will check your references, and, depending on the policy of the agency, you may have to take a drug test. The agency may or may not perform a criminal background check.

Employment agencies make money when you receive employment, so they tend to favor qualified candidates with some experience.

Federal and State Hiring Procedures

Federal and state institutions must follow certain regulations when hiring employees. State regulations vary by state. These regulations are designed to make the hiring process fair for everyone. Although most hospitals hire according to federal and state hiring guidelines, many small practices do not.

Federal and state hiring procedures help larger companies keep certain criteria in mind as they hire large numbers of people. Employment requirements are much stricter in federal and state owned and operated environments.

Examples of federal and state hiring procedures include:

▶ Companies must keep an application on active file for at least six months.
▶ Companies must clearly and adequately identify the requirements of a position in the vacancy announcement so that applicants understand the basis on which their application will be evaluated. This will also ensure that applicants possess the necessary skills to perform the work.
▶ Companies may not set standards for any job that adversely affect the hiring chances of any one group of people, and the standards must be job related, not person related. The Qualification Standards for General Schedule Positions, or X-188, describes the legal standards of various jobs.

▶ Companies must interview at least three to five people for the opening.

▶ Companies may not discriminate on the basis of race, religion, national origin, age, sex, marital status, or physical handicap.

▶ Any hiring tests must be related to the specific job for which the candidate has applied, and question responses may not reduce the chances of minorities, women, or a disproportionate number of candidates in any single group.

THE INSIDE TRACK

Who:	Aimee Davidson
What:	Dental Assistant I
How Long:	14 months
How Much:	$30,000 annual salary
Degree:	Three years of college
School:	University of Georgia, Central Piedmont Community College

INSIDER'S ADVICE

When I was growing up, I always said I wanted to be a dentist. Somewhere around high school and my first year of college, I changed my mind. I think when you are that young, the thought of going to school for eight years seems so long. Now that I am 26, I have realized eight years is a very small amount of time in the whole grand scheme of things. I wish I had followed my dream right after high school, because I would be graduating from dental school right now.

My advice is to follow your dream straight through to the end. Decide what type of job would make you happy, and go for it with the realization that you want more from life. When I interviewed for my job, I was the only one out of ten who didn't have experience. Dr. Welborne later told me that he would have hired me on the spot if I had had some experience. However, the other applicants may have had the experience, but they didn't have the personality he wanted. As a dental assistant, you sit only about a foot away from the doctor for almost eight hours a day. I showed him how serious I was about my dreams and this job, and he gave me the chance I feel I deserved and still work hard for.

INSIDER'S FUTURE

My goal is to become a dentist. I am currently working on completing my bachelor's degree. I used to take classes at night and work full time, but now I work about 30 hours a week and take one or two classes a semester during the day. You don't have to have a four-year degree to be accepted into dental school. There are general requirements to meet and a Dental Admissions Test to take. A four-year degree improves your chances of getting in. I plan to take the DAT in the fall of 1998 and will submit my application for dental school with the hope of being accepted for the fall of 1999.

CHAPTER **two**

ALL ABOUT TRAINING PROGRAMS

THIS CHAPTER is all about the training you need for your future in healthcare. It begins by explaining why you need to get training and reviews the types of training courses that are available. You will see several sample courses from training programs across the country, so you can get an idea of what types of programs and classes are offered for each job. Work study and internships are also discussed, as well as how to check to see whether a program is accredited. There are tips on studying for exams, taking notes, networking with classmates, getting to know your instructors, and using the career placement or counseling office in your chosen school. You will also find helpful sample interviews with employment recruiters, instructors, healthcare workers, and students who can give you the inside scoop.

WHY YOU NEED TRAINING

Most jobs in the healthcare field, especially those that involve direct patient treatment or the operation of equipment, will require a training period in a clinical setting to familiarize you with hospital or physician office procedures. Requirements for entering the field often include the completion of a training program that usually leads to some kind of certificate or associate degree.

You can find programs at technical schools or community colleges and certificates or degrees for almost every area of healthcare at different levels. A training program is worth considering if it is accredited, if you can commit to the time, and if the subject is one you want to pursue as a career. When you apply for a job, a degree or a certificate from a training program is a nice part of your application package that makes you more desirable to interviewers.

A hospital employment recruiter from Tampa, Florida, says:

> *Most hospitals will not hire someone without state certified training. We do not train individuals who do not have any experience because we have such a high volume of patients who need care. We need people who are familiar with their job and who meet the standards set by state or national certificate examinations. I would say 100 percent of the people we hire at our hospital have a certificate or degree of some kind, unless they are in a position such as housekeeping that does not require direct patient care.*

Making Decisions about Training

Deciding on the right training program may seem challenging since there are so many choices. Remember the personal evaluation you created in Chapter 1? Use that evaluation to consider the questions below. Though you may not know the answers right away, this checklist can help you decide which training program is right for you and allow you to focus your career goals.

▶ Do I need a job now or can I wait and gain greater experience through education?
▶ How long do I want to be in school before getting a job?
▶ Am I interested in work study or internships?
▶ What kind of financial aid can I receive from the school?
▶ Can I receive enough financial aid to attend a larger college or university?
▶ What school can I afford or be accepted to?
▶ How much will tuition, books, and tools cost?

Your budget and the cost of the training program will help determine whether you should work part time and go to school part time, apply for financial aid, or participate in work study, and whether you can afford an institute, a college, or a university. Another key consideration is whether or not you think you can meet the prerequisites and expectations of a particular program and will be accepted after you commit to the application process.

- What schools are in my area?
- Can I or do I want to relocate?
- Can I visit the school?
- What are the eligibility requirements for the program of study I would like to pursue?
- Have I completed or can I complete all program prerequisites?
- Do I have the aptitude to succeed?

You will also need to determine whether you can afford to relocate. A school may be in your state but not in your town. Can you afford moving expenses? Can you afford a place of your own? Does the school have dormitories where you may live at a lower price? (Most small schools don't.) If you want to attend an out-of-state school, you should expect your tuition to double. Before you apply to any school, be sure to visit and find out if it fits your needs.

- What kind of certification or degree do I want to complete?
- Would I rather train in a hospital, a private group practice, or a nursing home?
- Where do I want to work?
- What population do I want to help (children, adolescents, adults, seniors)?
- What salary range do I want?
- What sort of coworkers do I want?

These questions are very important because they will help determine what kind of job you will train for. You should research career options by visiting hospitals, physician practices, and other health organizations in your area to experience the work environment and meet some workers. If, for example, you discover through your personal research that you want to train and work in a hospital, you may not be interested in becoming a dental assistant.

While it is important to set goals for your career, be open to researching work environments that you might not originally have considered. Talk to people in the field. Try to get in touch with professional organizations to get a sense of the local professional community; many healthcare workers would be thrilled to speak with someone who might be interested in entering the field.

Also, there is no need to lock yourself into anything permanent after you finish one level of schooling. You may decide to further your education so you can reach a higher status and salary. Or after becoming, say, a pediatric medical assistant, you may find you do not work well with children and decide that you would rather work with adults. Keep an open mind and know that if one facet of healthcare is not a perfect fit for you, there might very well be another career in the field that will seem just right.

A registered nurse from Pompton Lakes, New Jersey, says:

> I was lucky I entered healthcare because I'm good at it. When I began as a nursing assistant, though, I didn't know that. I began in orthopedics and then decided pediatrics looked like fun. I tried being in the birthing room and didn't like it; then I tried taking care of the babies and didn't like that either. I had gone back to school and worked part time to become a registered nurse with an associate degree. I had a friend in the surgery recovery room, so I traded a shift with her to try that. I liked surgery, and I've been in here for fifteen years. Don't assume you will stay with what you have chosen. You may discover open roads once you're working.

Depending on the regulations of the state in which you live and the type of training program you are considering, certification is required for many, but not all, health careers. When you sign up for a particular training program, you will learn the requirements. Usually, after you graduate you will take the state or national certification examinations before going on to employment.

ENTRANCE REQUIREMENTS FOR TRAINING PROGRAMS

Depending on the program and school you attend, you may have to complete an entrance exam such as the *Science Placement Test* (SPT), the *Health Occupations Basic Entrance Test* (HOBET), or the *College Placement Test* (CPT) to determine your placement in courses. These tests evaluate your reading, writing, and math skills. For example, if you score low in math and high in science, you may be placed in a lower-level math course.

As an example, the HOBET measures competency in eight areas:

1. critical reading ability compared with the level necessary for college
2. basic math
3. reading speed of college-level material
4. reading rate and comprehension
5. test-taking skills
6. stress levels
7. social interaction
8. your most effective learning approach

The HOBET will not only identify your weaknesses in those processing skills necessary for success in college, but will also enable you to correct your weaknesses prior to entering school. The diagnostic report generated by the HOBET can alert both tutors and the college learning centers to your special needs, so that you can get assistance before you experience problems that may tarnish your academic record.

Some schools also require allied health entrance exams such as the *Allied Health Aptitude Test* (AHAT) for entrance into community college health-care programs and the *Allied Health Profession Aptitude Test* (AHPAT) for entrance into four-year colleges. These tests help identify qualified applicants by measuring general academic abilities and scientific knowledge.

The AHAT is a standardized test developed by the Psychological Association for use in determining the probable success of students applying for admission to undergraduate associate degree programs in allied health fields such as clinical laboratory technology, respiratory therapy, radiologic technology, and dental hygiene. It consists of four parts: quantitative reasoning, verbal reasoning, science knowledge, and reading ability.

The AHPAT is a standardized test developed by the Psychological Association for use in assessing the probable success of students applying for admission to bachelor's degree programs in allied health fields such as physical therapy, occupational therapy, medical technology, and physician's assistant. It consists of five parts: quantitative reasoning, verbal reasoning, biology, chemistry, and reading ability.

Other criteria used in admitting applicants to programs include the *Standard Achievement Test* (SAT), which you may be taking or have taken in high school, the *American College Test* (ACT), other reading, writing, or science placement tests, grade point average, recommendations and personal statements, and exams specific to certain fields, such as the *Nursing School Entrance Exam* (NSEE) or the *Pharmacy College Admissions Test* (PCAT). Current information on the PCAT is available at www.psychcorp.pearson assessments.com.

TYPES OF TRAINING

Educational requirements for the health occupations discussed in this book generally range from several month to one-year certificate programs to two years of college. Training for entry-level positions is offered in high schools, vocational-technical centers, community colleges, universities, hospitals, nursing homes, and the Armed Forces, depending on the type of program you are seeking. Most programs provide both classroom and clinical instruction, where you will actually get to work in a hospital, clinic, physician's office, or other healthcare environment. Many programs also offer opportunities for online or distance learning.

High School Programs for Nongraduated Students

If you have not yet graduated from high school or received your GED and you are under 20 years old, your area school district may have a youth apprenticeship program designed just for you. This type of program is also for high school students who want to pursue healthcare careers. Apprenticeship programs team with appropriate governmental and social service agencies to help students gain structured school- and work-based learning that can lead to a high school diploma, post-secondary credentials, or a certificate of occupational skills along with an introduction to the social skills and aptitudes needed for success in any job situation. Healthcare programs work with hospitals to open avenues to higher education and certifiable occupations, which will offer students better jobs with higher wages down the line when they are done with their training.

School districts offer other programs such as tech prep, cooperative education, internships, explorations in technology, and MicroSociety.

Tech prep programs are nationally recognized educational programs that enable students to receive community college credit for certain course-work they complete in high school. Tech prep programs almost always feature more supervised hands-on learning than traditional classroom instruction, and students have opportunities to develop the skills they will need on the job in the healthcare field.

Cooperative education is a structured method of combining classroom-based education with practical work experience. A cooperative education experience, commonly known as a *co-op*, provides academic credit for structured job experience.

Internships are jobs students take on in order to gain on-the-job experience in their chosen field. Internships may count toward course credit and may or may not be paid positions.

MicroSociety is a nonprofit organization that specializes in building motivating learning environments for students by bringing real life to learning. Although MicroSociety is primarily geared toward students in grades K-8, some school districts offer extended programming for high school study. Learn more at www.microsociety.org.

These examples may vary from state to state, but they all offer educational skills to apply in real-life healthcare employment situations. Call your local school district for more information.

Certificate Programs

Certificate programs are usually three-month to six-month or six-month to one-year programs, after which graduates receive a certificate of completion. Entrance requirements include a high school diploma or its equivalent. Entrance exams may be required. Courses combine classroom theory with clinical instruction. Certificate programs differ from college programs in that students attend the program straight through, with no breaks except holidays.

Every school's program has a different set of class names and descriptions, but the basic information you need to learn remains the same. As you can see from the tuition descriptions for each program listed below, being an in-state student is much easier on the wallet; the tuition doubles and sometimes triples for out-of-state students.

The three certificate training programs described below will give you an idea of what you can expect to find in a training program near you.

Nursing Assistant Sample Courses

Curriculum for certificate programs varies among schools and programs. For example, a one-quarter, three-month certificate course in a nursing assistant program from Big Bend Community College in Moses Lake, Washington, includes the following courses:

> **NUR 100, Nursing Assistant.** To prepare nursing assistants for competency as outlined by federal and Washington State curricula. Introduction to healthcare and nursing using classroom, laboratory, self-directed study, and observational experiences.
>
> **NUR 105, Nursing Trends Laboratory.** Taken concurrently with the nursing assistant core course. The campus laboratory is designed to allow the nursing student to gain proficiency in nursing skills prior to delivering nursing care within a healthcare facility.

As in many other training programs of this kind, the certificate requires only two classes, but the classes take up the whole quarter and are full time. The tuition is $73 per credit hour for in-state students and $215 per credit hour for out-of-state students. The program requires 70 to 80 hours total. A work-study program is provided.

At Saint Johns River Community College in Palatka, Florida, workforce education programs prepare graduates for immediate entry into the work force or give working individuals the chance to upgrade their skills. The Saint Johns Health-Sciences Building is a state-of-the-art facility that simulates a hospital setting. The nursing assistant program includes classes in the study of medical terminology, legal and ethical responsibilities, gerontology, nutrition, pet-facilitated therapy, and cardiopulmonary resuscitation (CPR) among other classes. Upon completion of the program, students are eligible to take the national nursing assistant exam to become certified (CNA.) The college also offers a Vocational Certificate in Nursing Assisting (Long-term Care).

Surgical Technician Sample Courses

The following course descriptions are from a one-year certificate program in surgical technology at Temple Junior College in Temple, Texas.

> **STTE 1301, Introduction to Surgical Technology.** Includes the history and legal aspects of surgery, psychology of adjustment, environmental control, patient care in preoperative, intraoperative, and postoperative periods.
> **STTE 1202, Surgical Terminology.** Analysis of basic work structure and development of a medical vocabulary related to the body and its systems.
> **STTE 1603, Human Structure and Function.** Structure and function of the human body with special emphasis on anatomical structures related to surgical intervention.

Tuition at Temple Community College is $75 per credit hour for in-state students and $120 per credit hour for out-of-state students. The total program requires 52 hours. (Program hour length varies by program and school.) Liability insurance is provided by the school. After graduation, students take the National Certified Exam to be certified as surgical technologists. This program is accredited by the CAAHEP. Some colleges also offer an associate degree for surgical technicians.

Dental Assistant Sample Courses

Here is a partial course description of a 12-month certificate program in dental assisting from Chemeketa Community College in Salem, Oregon.

BI060, Basic Science Principles. Designed for dental assisting and hospital systems management students. Presents introductory concepts of cell biology, microbiology, chemistry, and physics as applied to specific topics. Includes practical application of problem solving, scientific observation and measurement, use of equipment, and basic laboratory techniques.

DEN050, Dental Sciences I. A study of the sciences within the practice of dentistry. Includes oral microbiology, oral pathology, sterilization and disinfection principles, OSHA pathogens, anesthesia, dental office emergencies, and pharmacology.

DEN051, Introductory Concepts in Dental Assisting. Designed to introduce the student to basic general and oral anatomy. Particular attention directed toward physiological processes of the body, the oral cavity and its associated structures, and anatomical terminology.

Courses will vary by school and availability for the dental assisting program.

Tuition at Chemeketa Community College is $78 per hour for in-state students and $243 per hour for out-of-state students. However, after 90 days the tuition rate for out-of-state students drops to the same as for in-state students. The total program requires 52 hours. Liability insurance is provided by the school, and work study is available. Program graduates take the DANB examinations to be certified as dental assistants. This course is accredited by the ADA Commission. An associate degree in dental assisting is also available at many schools.

Associate Degree Programs

An associate degree program requires two academic or two calendar years. Entrance requirements include a high school diploma or a GED, and some programs require college prep courses. Most associate degree programs require entrance and placement exams. In an associate degree program, half the required courses are in liberal arts and half are in the specific major. Courses in the major combine classroom theory with clinical practice in extended care facilities, hospitals, urgent care clinics, and community agencies.

The benefit of receiving a two-year associate degree is the combination of liberal arts classes with medical classes, as well as the opportunity for a better job and higher pay. In addition, colleges offer clubs and organizations that offer students valuable life experience. While attending a college, participate in as many campus activities as you can rather than restricting yourself to activities related to your major.

One nursing student from Orlando, Florida, shares some advice:

> *The best thing I ever did was take an acting class. I know acting doesn't have anything to do with being a nursing assistant, but it gave me an outlet so I didn't feel confined to biology and labs. I didn't want my whole school career to be nursing, but I knew I wouldn't become a famous actress either. I met some interesting people, and the class was a lot of fun. The acting class gave me a break from the daily routine of health and also helped me as I trained to work with people.*

Radiologic Technician Sample Courses

A radiologic technician associate degree from Athens Technical Institute in Athens, Georgia, requires the following types of courses:

General Education

ENG 191, Composition and Rhetoric. Expository themes in both general and medical topics developed by basic rhetorical methods. Effective writing techniques.

MAT 191, College Algebra. A study of algebra, including absolute values and inequalities; complex numbers; functions including polynomial, rational, exponential, and logarithmic functions; systems of equations; and the binomial theorem.

Radiologic Technology Major

RAD 101, Introduction to Radiography. Provides an overview of radiography, patient care, and the profession as a whole with emphasis on patient care, considering both physical and psychological conditions. Topics include ethics, medical and legal consideration, professionalism, basic principles of radiation protection, basic principles of exposure, equipment, hospital and departmental organizations, body mechanics, vital signs, medical emergencies, contrast agents, CPR, and death and dying.

RAD 107, Principles of Radiographic Exposure I. Introduces factors that govern and influence the production of the radiographic image on radiographic film. Lab demonstrations. Topics include radiographic density, contrast, recorded detail, distortion, exposure latitude, film holders, processing, handling and storage, and state and federal regulations.

Courses will vary by school, semester, and availability for an associate degree in radiologic technology.

At Athens Technical Institute, students pay $58 per credit hour. The radiology technician associate degree requires 139 hours total. Insurance is provided by the school, and graduates are eligible to sit for the National Certification Examination (NCE). The program is accredited by the Joint Review Committee on Education in Radiologic Technology (JRCERT).

Medical Assistant Sample Courses

An example of the course curriculum for an associate degree in medical assisting from Pitt Community College in Greenville, North Carolina, follows:

General Education

CAS 100, Introduction to Microcomputer Applications. General introduction to the microcomputer, DOS, and various software application packages, including word processing, spreadsheets, and database management.

OSC 110, Word Processing. Software program developed for use on the MS-DOS microcomputer. Designed to give the student a basic understanding of the WP software and the operation and application of the microcomputer through classroom instruction and hands-on experience.

Medical Assisting Major

BIO 101, Basic Anatomy and Physiology. Foundation of facts and principles in the normal structure and related functioning of the following body systems: skeletal, muscular, digestive, circulatory, respiratory, urinary, reproductive, endocrine, integumentary, nervous, and special sense organs. Presents principles and concepts of physiology and immunology.

BIO 101A, Basic Anatomy and Physiology Laboratory. Laboratory setting presents the student with a foundation of facts and principles in the normal structure and related functioning of the human body.

Courses will vary by school, semester, and availability.

Tuition at Pitt Community College is $50 per credit hour for in-state students and $241 per credit hour for out-of-state students. The program requires 109 hours total. Malpractice insurance is available from the school, and work study is available. After graduation, students are required to complete an application to the AAMA to take the Medication Aide/Assistant Certification Examination (MACE) to become CMAs. A certificate course is also available at some schools for the medical assistant program.

Physical Therapy Assistant Sample Courses

Here is a sampling of the course curriculum of the physical therapy assistant program at Volunteer State Community College in Gallatin, Tennessee:

General Education

ENG101, Composition and Rhetoric. Emphasizes the development and improvement of written and oral communication abilities.

MAT131, College Algebra. Emphasizes problem solving techniques. Topics include fundamental algebra concepts and operations, linear and quadratic equations and functions, simultaneous equations, inequalities, exponents and powers, graphing techniques, and word problems.

Physical Therapy Assistant Major

BIO231, Human Anatomy and Physiology I. Introduces the structure and function of the body as a whole and studies of the integumentary (skin), skeletal, muscular, nervous, sensory, and endocrine systems.

BIO232, Human Anatomy and Physiology II. Studies the structure and function of the following body systems: blood, lymphatic, cardiovascular, respiratory, digestive, urinary, and reproductive. The student will also be introduced to metabolism, nutrition, and heredity.

PTA110, Physical Science for the Physical Therapy Assistant. Focuses on basic, normal structure and function of the human body. Topics include an overview of each body system and how systems coordinate activities to maintain a balanced state, recognizing deviations from the normal.

Courses will vary by school, semester, and availability.

Tuition at Volunteer State Community College is $48 per credit hour for in-state students and $190 per credit hour for out-of-state students. The program requires 109 hours total. Malpractice insurance is available through the school. Graduates are required to pass the appropriate state examinations for a physical therapy assistant license. This course is accredited by the Committee on Accreditation for Physical Therapy Education (CAPTE).

Baccalaureate Programs

The baccalaureate program, or bachelor's degree program, combines courses within your desired major with general education in a four-year curriculum in a college or university. You may be admitted to your major program as a freshman or after one or two years of general education or liberal arts courses. If you go to a small college or technical school to become a surgical technician with an associate degree, and then decide after about a year that you want to move on to a higher degree and level of salary, you can always go back to school to obtain a bachelor's degree as long as you complete the coursework required by your chosen college or university.

A high school diploma or a GED is required for admission, and placement exams, SAT scores, ACT scores, and an acceptable high school GPA (grade point average) may be required. Entrance requirements may be more competitive than for shorter training programs. To enter the specific major area, you may be required to take a higher level of tests, such as the AHAT or the DAT. A bachelor's degree requires at least four years of school if you do not already have some schooling. Like most students, you may therefore require some financial aid.

Attending college for several years is not for everyone, so be sure that the health occupation you choose doesn't require more training than you are willing to commit yourself to. On the other hand, do not immediately write off a college education for financial reasons. Remember, there are scholarships and loans, plus a number of other ways to help pay for college. (See Chapter 4 for details about financial aid.)

Work Study Programs

Regardless of which training program you select, you should consult your career counselor or advisor to see if your school has a work study program. Work study programs provide assistance for full-time students who need additional financial aid by giving them first priority to take on-campus or on-site jobs in order to subsidize their tuition and/or earn living money while in college. Work hours—no more than 20 hours per week—do not compete with class hours, and students gain extra work experience in the process. Work study programs are provided on the basis of need. If you elect to use this option to subsidize your time in school, look at it as having a leg up on your peers—you gain on-the-job experience in addition to your classes, without the burden of long hours. This is a great way to experience a professional work environment and the associated responsibilities.

Internships

One of the best ways to gain practical job skills is through an internship in which you can experience a professional work environment in your chosen field. To begin your search for an internship, consult your school's career development, counseling, or internship offices. Let your counselor know the ideal type of experience you are seeking. If you are looking for a paid internship, your choices will be significantly fewer; most internships are unpaid. Remember that the experience you gain could lead to a full-time position, making an unpaid internship well worth your time.

Companies across the nation provide internships for prospective healthcare students. For example, the American Heart Association offers a variety of summer internship programs, as well as one-semester and one-year terms. The internships are offered nationwide, and grants are available as well. The March of Dimes offers a flexible number of part-time and year-round internships. Many other organizations offer internships, including the Leukemia Society of America, the American Cancer Society, the American Red Cross, and other smaller companies like Action AIDS. For more information on these associations, talk to your counselor and see the Appendix under Internships.

Training via the Armed Forces

The military provides training and work experience in healthcare and many other fields for more than 1.5 million people who serve in the active Army, Navy, Marine Corps, Air Force, and Coast Guard, their reserve components, and the Air and Army National Guard. In order to join the services, you must sign a legal agreement called an enlistment contract, which usually involves a commitment to eight years of service. Depending on the terms of the contract, two to six years are spent on active duty and the balance is spent in the reserves. The enlistment contract obligates the military to provide the agreed-upon job, rating, pay, cash bonuses for enlistment in certain occupations, medical and other benefits, occupational training, and continuing education. In return, enlisted personnel must serve satisfactorily for the period specified.

Requirements for each service vary, but certain qualifications for enlistment are common to all branches. In order to enlist, you must be between 17 and 35 years old, be a U.S. citizen or immigrant alien holding permanent resident status, not have a felony record, and possess a birth certificate. Applicants who are aged 17 must have the consent of a parent or legal guardian before entering the service. Coast Guard enlisted personnel must enter active duty before their 28th birthday, while Marine Corps enlisted personnel must not be over 29. Applicants must both pass a written examination—the Armed Services Vocational Aptitude Battery (ASVAB)—and meet certain minimum physical standards such as height, weight, vision, and overall health. All branches of the Armed Forces require high school graduation or its equivalent for certain enlistment options.

People thinking about enlisting in the military should learn as much as they can about military life before making a decision. This is especially important if you are thinking about making the military a career. Speaking to friends and relatives with military experience is a good idea. Determine what the military can offer you and what it will expect in return. Then, talk to a recruiter, who can determine whether you qualify for enlistment, explain the various enlistment options, and tell you which military occupational specialties currently have openings.

Ask the recruiter for the branch you have chosen to assess your chances of being accepted for training in the occupation of your choice, or, better still, take the aptitude exam to see how well you score. The military uses the aptitude exam as a placement exam, and test scores largely determine an individual's chances of being accepted into a particular training program. Selection for a particular type of training depends on the needs of the service, your general and technical aptitudes, and your personal preference. Because all prospective recruits are required to take the exam, those who do so before committing themselves to enlist have the advantage of knowing in advance whether they stand a good chance of being accepted for training in a particular specialty.

If you decide to join the military, the next step is to pass the physical examination and sign the enlistment contract. Negotiating the contract involves choosing, qualifying, and agreeing on a number of enlistment options such as length of active duty time, which may vary according to the enlistment option.

All services offer a delayed entry program, by which an individual may delay entry into active duty for up to one year after enlisting. High school students may enlist during their senior year and enter a service after graduation. Others choose this program because the job training they desire is not currently available but will be within the coming year, or because they need time to arrange personal affairs.

Women are eligible to enter most military specialties (for example, mechanic, missile maintenance technician, heavy equipment operator, and fighter pilot, as well as medical care, administrative support, and intelligence specialties). Generally, only occupations involving direct exposure to combat are excluded.

People planning to apply the skills gained through military training to a civilian career should first determine how good the prospects are for civilian employment in jobs related to the military specialty that interests them. Second, they should know the prerequisites for the related civilian job. Because many civilian occupations require a license, certification, or minimum level of education, it is important to determine whether military training is sufficient to enter the civilian equivalent or, if not, what additional training will be required.

Many service people get college credit for the technical training they receive on duty, which, combined with off-duty courses, can lead to an associate degree through community college programs such as the Community College of the Air Force. In addition to on-duty training, military personnel may choose from a variety of educational programs. Most military installations have tuition assistance programs for people wishing to take courses during off-duty hours.

In addition to basic pay, military personnel receive free room and board (or a tax-free housing and subsistence allowance), medical and dental care, a military clothing allowance, military supermarket and department store shopping privileges, 30 days of paid vacation a year (referred to as *leave*), and travel opportunities. In many duty stations, military personnel may receive a housing allowance that can be used for off-base housing. Other allowances are paid for foreign duty, hazardous duty, submarine and flight duty, and employment as a medical officer. Athletic and other facilities—such as gymnasiums, tennis courts, golf courses, bowling centers, libraries, and movie theaters—are available on many military installations. Military personnel are eligible for retirement benefits after 20 years of service.

Each of the military services publishes handbooks, factsheets, and pamphlets describing entrance requirements, training and advancement opportunities, and other aspects of a military career. These publications are widely available at all recruiting stations, at most state employment service offices, high schools, colleges, public libraries, and on the web at www.bls.gov/oco/ ocos249.htm. Information on educational and other veterans' benefits is available from VA (Veterans Administration) offices located throughout the country.

CHOOSING THE RIGHT TRAINING PROGRAM

Before you begin the application process, you should find out all you can about the school(s) you want to attend. Applying can be a very time-consuming and costly process, so finding out the details up front will save you time, money, and energy in the long run. Here are some important questions to ask about each training program:

► **What requirements must I meet?** You may be required to take a certain number of English, math, or science courses or comparable placement tests to be considered for your training program. You may also need to take the SAT or ACT if you have not already taken one of these in high school.

► **Is the program I'm interested in accredited? By whom?** Accreditation is very important; it tells you the school offers high-quality education. Many agencies accredit programs in every field of the healthcare industry. Do not be overwhelmed by the number of accrediting associations. Just be sure your targeted school lists one or more of them as its accrediting agency.

For example, the Curriculum Review Board (CRB) of the AAMA assesses the quality of programs seeking accreditation for medical assistant technology. It then advises the Council on Accreditation and Unit Recognition (CAUR) CAAHEP as to whether the program should be accredited.

CAAHEP and ABHES are both recognized by the U.S. Department of Education for accrediting such programs. For a list of associations that maintain lists or directories on accredited programs, see the Appendix under Accrediting Agencies.

▶ **What are the faculty members' qualifications and experience?** The program should include some faculty members with advanced degrees (MS, MBA, PhD, JD, and so on) and some with significant experience in the working world (at least five to seven years). The faculty should be accessible for one-on-one student conferences. To get a sense of how often students interact with faculty, visit the campus and try to speak to some current students.

▶ **What percentage of graduates were placed in jobs upon graduation? Is there a career placement office or a counselor/advisor on campus?** The placement rate for graduates is extremely important, and when considering a school, whether small or large, you should ask about it. Many schools offer free placement services for the working lifetime of their graduates.

▶ **Is the school equipped with the latest technology?** Again, always visit the school you plan to attend, and ask to see the laboratory facilities and equipment. The most recent and advanced computer technology and training equipment should be available to students.

Tips on Applying to Programs

▶ Apply as early as you can. You'll need to fill out an application and submit official high school or GED transcripts and any copies of SAT, ACT, or other test scores used for admission. If you have not taken these, you will have to take them before you can be admitted. Call the school and find out when the next programs starts, then apply at least a month or two prior to that date to make sure you can complete the requirements before the program starts.

▶ With your application, you will receive a prewritten request for transcripts from the admissions office. Make sure you send out those requests as soon as possible, so the admissions process is not held up in any way.

▶ Make the earliest possible appointment to take any placement tests that may be required, so as not hold up admissions.

▶ Pay your fees before the deadline. Enrollment is not complete each quarter or semester until the student has paid all fees by the date specified on the registration form. If fees are not paid by the deadline, the classes will be canceled. If you are going to receive financial aid, apply as early as you can to avoid fee default.

▶ Find out whether you must pass a physical or submit any other medical history forms on file for the school you choose, so as not to hold up admissions.

MAKING THE MOST OF A TRAINING PROGRAM

After you have done your research, gone through the application process, waited for a response, made your final decision, paid your first bills, and finally entered a training program to receive a certificate or degree, you want to make the most of your training experience, right? The rest of this chapter shows you how to maximize the learning process. Apply the tips listed below to get the most out of your training program.

How to Study for Exams

Remember studying for exams in high school? No matter how extensive your background or how well you did in high school, studying is crucial to success in a specialized training program, where the work is much tougher than in high school. But do not let the word *exam* make you nervous. Exams are the instructor's way of finding out what you have learned and what you may need to review before going any further with assignments. The major difference is that in a healthcare training program, it is important that you recall the techniques you learn and will be able to apply the experience to real life.

A radiology instructor from Athens Technical Institute in Athens, Georgia, says:

> *Some of the rad tech program involves reviewing the anatomy you have to demonstrate on radiograms. Some is positioning. Some studying is*

strictly academic, such as going over your notes from class, reading the chapter, and writing down key points. Studying depends mostly on the type of course you have. We have labs that review much of the information learned in class. However, learning anatomy requires memorization, and if you're not good at memorization, you may have to study more than others do.

Some instructors will tell you to study at least two hours for each hour of class. This may seem difficult and time-consuming, but there are ways to make it easier, including reviewing your notes, reading appropriate textbook chapters, studying with others, and studying between classes.

If you remain on task in classes and labs, and review steadily, you should have no problem with exams. Many exams are multiple choice and the wrong answer choices will point you to the correct answer. Essay exams require you to write more information than a regular multiple choice test can ask for. Your instructor may let you know what format he or she will use, so you can study accordingly. During the test, remember to read the instructions carefully and listen to your instructor's directions.

How to Take Notes in Class

Taking good notes in class will help you to study after class. Listen attentively and try to write down the most important information. Many instructors will indicate what you should write down and what is already in the book you will be studying. If an instructor writes anything on the board or on an overhead, you should write it too. Writing down too much information is better than writing too little, but be sure you are listening to the instructor as well as taking notes.

A medical assistant instructor from Santa Barbara Business School, Santa Barbara, California, says:

The problem most students have is they try to write down everything that's said, a laundry list of things. What they need to do is listen for key points and concepts, and the textbook will have all the little details that they can go back and read. It's a good idea to read the chapter before you come to class, so you know what's in there and have questions ready for the instructor. And supplement your note-taking. Make a note about something you didn't understand well when you read it or be prepared to ask questions that could set the tone for the lecture.

Rewriting your notes from each class helps you sort out the needed information and helps reinforce the information discussed in class.

Studying with Other Students

Studying with other students is one of the best ways to learn. Teaching another person can help you to learn and remember the material. It is a good way to identify any gaps in your knowledge. Also, having someone quiz you or explain something that you do not understand makes the information more real and dynamic. Create a study group or join one, and together with classmates massage your knowledge of your particular program.

An Athens, Georgia, resident radiology instructor says:

We have small, limited classes, so we try to pick people we feel will best succeed. They shouldn't be competitive but should be supportive of each other. Small study groups really help reinforce things. Another thing we do is labs, where students position each other like patients in the hospital. Basically, they have to work together, interacting in the clinic and labs, so they get to know each other and have their own war stories to tell each other. Study groups are really a good idea.

Also, in case you did not take very good notes or missed a day of class, your fellow students' notes may help you catch up. Of course, you should not miss any classes if you can possibly help it.

Getting to Know Your Instructor

The first thing you should do after entering a class is make an appointment to meet with the instructor so you can ask questions, get to know him or her, and find out what is expected of you. Each instructor is different and has different expectations. Also, if you have a child at home or some problem that might take time away from the class, you can inform the instructor ahead of time.

In the clinical classes, you may have the opportunity to get to know instructors personally while working directly with them. Many instructors work one-on-one with students in the most difficult part of the program to make sure they understand the procedures and instructions, become oriented, and really learn that procedure. Instructors may go with you to the hospital or clinic where you will receive additional clinical education.

Using the Career Planning and Placement Office

Most schools have a career planning and placement office. Make an appointment right away to meet with a counselor in your field so you can begin working on a plan for job hunting before your graduation or certificate release. Your counselor will help you build your resume, tell you about job prospects in your area of specialization, and perhaps set up a placement file that allows you to send resume information directly from the school.

Career centers offer a variety of career-advising activities, such as one-on-one sessions in which students and advisors discuss effective career decision-making preferences, interests, values, and other concerns. Establishing goals is an important part of these sessions. You can make an appointment at any time throughout your training program if you have questions about your future career. Other services offered may include a career services library, a videotape library, a Career and Life Development workshop, other workshops, an information line/job vacancy hotline, internship programs, student employment services, career days, and mock and on-campus interviews. Each school is different, so career placement programs and services will vary.

A career planning and placement counselor in New Orleans, Louisiana, has this advice:

> *The Career Planning and Placement Center is our way of reaching out to assist you in your search for suitable employment. How much*

you benefit from our services is up to you and your desire to find a career that fits your personality, abilities, and skills. Many people get stuck in a job they don't like because they didn't take the time to research the job. Make the career center at your school of choice one of your primary resources as you move toward your career goals. If you don't take advantage of your school's career placement service, you may wind up paying large fees to a private employment agency after you graduate.

THE INSIDE TRACK

Who:	Lisa Williams
What:	Medical technologist
Where:	Summit Medical Center, Frisco, Colorado
How Long:	Two years
How Much:	$30,000 annual salary
Degree:	Bachelor's degree in medical technology
School:	Medical College of Georgia, Augusta, Georgia

INSIDER'S ADVICE

I knew I wanted to do something in the medical field, and I knew nursing was not really up my alley. I called and requested information from medical schools around Georgia and read about the programs they offered. When I read about the medical technologist degree, I knew that was what I wanted to do. I could learn about five different lab areas without having to specialize in only one of them. The areas I work in are hematology, chemistry, microbiology, immunology, and blood bank.

Because I wasn't sure what I wanted to do, I researched my options. I found an accredited program and pursued my future career. Deciding on a career is not easy, but once you find something you like, stick with it and work hard. I decided to get my bachelor's degree because I had the time, and I received financial aid grants and loans to help with expenses. I am currently finishing paying off my student loans, and I am happy about the way I made my career decision.

INSIDER'S FUTURE

I plan to go back to school soon. I would like to one day receive my PhD, but I haven't decided in which field. It will either be immunology or pathology. I'm looking at another four to six years of school. I'm not sure where I will attend school because I would still like to move back to Georgia, where my family lives; I will have to research more schools. My ideal future job would be working as a doctor for the Center for Disease Control in Atlanta, helping to discover cures.

CHAPTER three

DIRECTORY OF HEALTHCARE TRAINING PROGRAMS

THIS CHAPTER contains a directory of technical and career schools, proprietary and vocational schools, independent colleges, and other schools that offer training programs for the healthcare jobs discussed in this book. Each entry gives the school name, address, and phone number, so you can contact any school directly to get more information as well as application forms for the programs that interest you.

ONCE YOU have decided to get into a training program, you need to find one at a school near you. First locate the job title you want, and then look under the state to find the schools in that area. The schools are listed in alphabetical order by city within each state, so you can quickly locate schools in nearby cities. Although the schools included in this chapter are not endorsed or recommended by LearningExpress®, this list is intended to help you begin your search for an appropriate school by offering a representative listing of accredited schools in each state. Since so many schools offer these programs, not all could be listed here because of space limitations. However, this representative listing should get you started. The Appendix includes names of professional associations you can contact for additional lists of accredited training programs in your area.

DENTAL ASSISTANT TECHNOLOGY

ALABAMA

Fortis College—Mobile
3590 Pleasant Valley Rd.
Mobile, AL 36609
334-953-6436

ARIZONA

Apollo College—Tri City, Inc.
630 W Southern Ave.
Mesa, AZ 85210
602-831-6585

Apollo College—Phoenix, Inc.
8503 N 27th Ave.
Phoenix, AZ 85015
602-864-1571

The Bryman School—Phoenix
2250 W Peoria Ave.
Ste. A-100
Phoenix, AZ 85029
877-431-8909

The Laural School
2538 N 8th St.
Phoenix, AZ 85006
602-947-6565

Apollo College
3870 N Oracle Rd.
Tucson, AZ 85705
520-888-5885

CALIFORNIA

National Education Center—Bryman
  Campus
1120 N Brookhurst St.
Anaheim, CA 92801
714-778-6500

Southern California College of Medical-
  Dental Care
1717 S Brookhurst St.
Anaheim, CA 92804
714-635-3450

San Joaquin Valley College
201 New Stine Rd.
Bakersfield, CA 93309
805-834-0126

Orange Coast College
2701 Fairview Rd.
Costa Mesa, CA 92626
714-432-0202

Galen College of Medical and Dental
  Assistants
1325 N Wishon Ave.
Fresno, CA 93728
559-264-9700

San Joaquin Valley College
3333 N Bond Ave.
Fresno, CA 93726
209-229-7800

Citrus College
1000 W Foothill Blvd.
Glendora, CA 91741
818-914-8516

Huntington College of Dental Technology
7466 Edinger Ave.
Huntington Beach, CA 92647
714-841-9500

National Education Center—Bryman
   Campus
5350 Atlantic Ave.
Long Beach, CA 90805
310-422-6007

Donald Vocational School
1833 W 8th St.
Los Angeles, CA 90057
310-483-2080

National Education Center—Bryman
   Campus
1017 Wilshire Blvd.
Los Angeles, CA 90017
213-481-1640

Nova Institute of Health Technology
2400 S Western Ave.
Los Angeles, CA 90018
213-735-2222

Galen College of Medical and Dental
   Assistants
1604 Ford Ave.
Modesto, CA 95350
209-527-5084

Concorde Career Institute
4150 Lankershim Blvd.
N Hollywood, CA 91602
818-766-8151

Nova Institute of Health Technology
520 N Euclid Ave.
Ontario, CA 91762
909-984-5027

Institute of Business and Medical
   Technology
75-110 St. Charles Pl.
Palm Desert, CA 92260
619-776-5873

Diablo Valley College
321 Golf Club Rd.
Pleasant Hill, CA 94523
510-685-1230

National Education Center—Bryman
   Campus
3505 N Hart Ave.
Rosemead, CA 91770
818-573-5470

Concorde Career Institute
570 W 4th St.
San Bernardino, CA 92401
909-884-8891

Concorde Career Institute
123 Camino De La Reina
San Diego, CA 92108
619-688-0800

National Education Center—Bryman
   Campus
731 Markey St.
San Francisco, CA 94103
415-777-2500

Concorde Career Institute
1290 N 1st St.
San Jose, CA 92108
408-441-6411

Western Career College
170 Bay Fair Mall
San Leandro, CA 94578
510-278-3888

Allan Hancock College
800 S College Dr.
Santa Maria, CA 93454
805-922-6966

Santa Rosa Junior College
1501 Mendocino Ave.
Santa Rosa, CA 95401
707-527-4100

Concorde Career Institute
6850 Van Nuys Blvd.
Van Nuys, CA 91405
818-780-5252

Galen College of Medical and Dental
   Assistants
3908 W Caldwell
Visalia, CA 93277
559-732-5200

San Joaquin Valley College
8400 W Mineral King Ave.
Visalia, CA 93291
559-651-2500

Nova Institute of Health Technology
11416 Whittier Rd.
Whittier, CA 90601
213-695-0771

National Education Center—Bryman
   Campus
20835 Sherman Way
Winnetka, CA 91306
818-887-7911

COLORADO

Concorde Career Institute
770 Grant St.
Denver, CO 80203
303-861-1151

Heritage College of Health Careers
12 Lakeside Ln.
Denver, CO 80212
303-477-7240

Front Range Community College
3645 W 112th Ave.
Westminster, CO 80030
303-466-8811

CONNECTICUT

Huntington Institute, Inc.
193 Broadway
Norwich, CT 06360
203-886-0507

FLORIDA

Concorde Career Institute
7960 Arlington Expwy.
Jacksonville, FL 32211
904-725-0525

Florida Community College at Jacksonville
501 W State St.
Jacksonville, FL 32202
904-632-3000

Palm Beach Community College
4200 Congress Ave.
Lake Worth, FL 33461
407-967-7222

Southern College
5600 Lake Underhill Rd.
Orlando, FL 32807
407-273-1000

Concorde Career Institute
4202 W Spruce St.
Tampa, FL 33607
813-874-0094

GEORGIA

Albany Technical Institute
1021 Lowe Rd.
Albany, GA 31708
912-430-3520

Atlanta College of Medical Dental Careers
1240 W Peachtree St. NE
Atlanta, GA 30309
404-249-8200

Medix Schools
2480 Windy Hill Rd.
Marietta, GA 30067
770-980-0002

IDAHO

American Institute of Health Technology, Inc.
1200 N Liberty St.
Boise, ID 83704
208-377-8080

ILLINOIS

Kaskaskia College
27210 College Rd.
Centralia, IL 62801
618-532-1981

Parkland College
2400 W Bradley Ave.
Champaign, IL 61821
217-351-2200

VIP Schools, Inc.
600 N McClurg Ct.
Chicago, IL 60611-3044
312-266-1484

INDIANA

Indiana University—Purdue University at
    Indianapolis, IN
355 N Lansing
Indianapolis, IN 46202
317-274-5555

Professional Career Institute
2611 Waterfront Pkwy., East Dr.
Indianapolis, IN 46214
317-299-6001

KANSAS

Bryan Institute
1004 S Oliver
Wichita, KS 67218
316-685-2284

LOUISIANA

Domestic Health Care Institute
4826 Jamestown Ave.
Baton Rouge, LA 70808
504-925-5312

Delta Schools, Inc.
4549 Johnston Dr.
Lafayette, LA 70503
318-988-2211

Eastern College of Health Vocation
3540 I-10 Service Rd. S
Metairie, LA 70001
504-834-8644

Delta Schools, Inc.
413 W Admiral Doyle
New Iberia, LA 70560
318-365-7348

MARYLAND

Medix Schools
1017 York Rd.
Towson, MD 21204
410-337-5155

MASSACHUSETTS

National Education Center—Bryman
Campus
323 Boylston St.
Brookline, MA 02146
617-232-6035

MICHIGAN

Ross Medical Education Center
4741 Washtenaw
Ann Arror, MI 48108
734-434-7320

Ferris State University
901 S State St.
Big Rapids, MI 49307
616-592-2100

Ross Medical Education Center
3630 Miller Rd., Ste. D
Flint, MI 48504
810-733-7488

Grand Rapids Community College
143 Bostwick Ave. NE
Grand Rapids, MI 49505
616-771-4000

Grand Rapids Educational Center
1750 Woodworth St. NE
Grand Rapids, MI 49505
616-364-8464

Ross Medical Education Center
1188 N West Ave.
Jackson, MI 49202
517-782-7677

Ross Medical Education Center
4106 West Jaginaw Hwy.
Lansing, MI 48917
517-703-9044

Ross Medical Education Center
6235 S. Westridge
Portage, MI 94002
810-758-7200

Ross Medical Education Center
950 Norton Ave., Ste. D
Roosevelt Park, MI 49441
231-729-1531

Ross Medical Education Center
4300 Fashion Square Blvd.
Saginaw, MI 48603
989-791-5792

Delta College
University Center, MI 48710
517-686-9000

MINNESOTA

Range Technical College—Hibbing Campus
2900 E Beltline
Hibbing, MN 55746
218-262-7200

Concorde Career Institute, Inc.
12 N 12th St.
Minneapolis, MN 55403
612-341-3850

Lakeland Medical and Dental Academy
1402 W Lake St.
Minneapolis, MN 55408
612-827-5656

Northeast Metro Technical College
3300 Century Ave. N
White Bear Lake, MN 55110
612-779-5827

MISSISSIPPI

Hinds Community College—Raymond
  Campus
Raymond, MS 39154
601-857-3212

MISSOURI

Concorde Career Institute
3239 Broadway
Kansas City, MO 64111
816-531-5223

Al-Med Academy
10963 St. Charles Rock Rd.
Saint Louis, MO 63074
314-739-4450

Missouri School for Doctors' Assistants
10121 Manchester Rd.
Saint Louis, MO 63122
314-821-7700

St. Louis Community College—Forest Park
5600 Oakland Ave.
Saint Louis, MO 63110
314-644-9280

NEVADA

American Academy for Career Education
3120 E Desert Inn Rd.
Las Vegas, NV 89121
702-732-7748

Professional Careers
3305 Spring Mountain Rd.
Las Vegas, NV 89120
702-368-2338

NEW HAMPSHIRE
New Hampshire Technical Institute
11 Institute Dr.
Concord, NH 03301
603-225-1865

NEW JERSEY
Camden County College
P.O. Box 200
Blackwood, NJ 08012
609-228-7200

Empire Technical School of New Jersey
576 Central Ave.
E Orange, NJ 07018
201-675-0565

Berdan Institute
265 Rte. 46 W
Totowa, NJ 07512
201-256-3444

NEW YORK
New York School for Medical and Dental
  Assistants
116-16 Queens Blvd.
Forest Hills, NY 11375
718-793-2330

Mandl School
254 W 54th St.
New York, NY 10019
212-247-3434

Techno-Dent Training Center
101 W 31st St.
New York, NY 10001
212-695-1818

Continental Dental Assistant School
633 Jefferson Rd.
Rochester, NY 14623
716-272-8060

NORTH CAROLINA
Alamance Community College
P.O. Box 8000
Graham, NC 27253
919-578-2002

Guilford Technical Community College
P.O. Box 309
Jamestown, NC 27282
919-334-4822

OHIO
Akron Medical-Dental Institute
733 W Market St.
Akron, OH 44303
216-762-9788

Institute of Medical-Dental Technology
375 Glensprings Dr.
Cincinnati, OH 45246
513-851-8500

Cleveland Institute of Dental-Medical
  Assistants
1836 Euclid Ave.
Cleveland, OH 44115
216-241-2930

Eastland Career Center
4465 S Hamilton Rd.
Groveport, OH 43125
614-836-3903

Cleveland Institute of Dental-Medical
   Assistants
5564 Mayfield Rd.
Lyndhurst, OH 44124
216-473-6273

Cleveland Institute of Dental-Medical
   Assistants
5733 Hopkins Rd.
Mentor, OH 44060
216-946-9530

OKLAHOMA

Metro Tech Vocational Technical Center
1900 Springlake Dr.
Oklahoma City, OK 73111
405-424-8324

Kiamichi AVTS SD #7—Talihina Campus
Rte. 2 & Hwy. 63A, P.O. Box 1800
Talihina, OK 74571
918-567-2264

Bryan Institute
2843 E 51st St.
Tulsa, OK 74105
918-749-6891

OREGON

Lane Community College
4000 E 30th Ave.
Eugene, OR 97405
503-747-4501

Apollo College—Portland, Inc.
2600 SE 98th Ave.
Portland, OR 97266
503-761-6100

College of America
921 SW Washington
Portland, OR 97205
503-242-9000

Portland Community College
P.O. Box 19000
Portland, OR 97280
503-244-6111

PENNSYLVANIA

Academy of Medical Arts and Business
279 Boas St.
Harrisburg, PA 17102
717-233-2172

Career Training Academy
703 5th Ave.
New Kensington, PA 15068
412-337-1000

Community College of Philadelphia
1700 Spring Garden St.
Philadelphia, PA 19130
215-715-8000

Delaware Valley Academy of Medical and
   Dental Assistants
3330 Grant Ave.
Philadelphia, PA 19149
215-676-1200

Median School of Allied Health Careers
125 7th St.
Pittsburgh, PA 15222
800-570-0693

RHODE ISLAND

Community College of Rhode Island
400 East Ave.
Warwick, RI 02886
401-825-1000

TENNESSEE

Chattanooga State Technical Community
   College
4501 Amnicola Hwy.
Chattanooga, TN 37406
615-697-4401

Memphis Area Vocational-Technical School
550 Alabama Ave.
Memphis, TN 38105-3799
901-543-6100

Shelbyville State Area Vocational Technical
   School
1405 Madison St.
Shelbyville, TN 37160
615-685-5013

TEXAS

Bryan Institute
1719 Pioneer Pkwy. W
Arlington, TX 76013
817-265-5588

Allied Health Careers
5424 Hwy. 290 W
Austin, TX 78735
512-892-5210

ATI Health Education Center
8150 Brookriver Dr.
Dallas, TX 75247
214-637-0980

Career Centers of Texas El Paso, Inc.
8375 Burnham Dr.
El Paso, TX 79907
915-595-1935

ATI Health Education Center
1200 Summit Ave.
Fort Worth, TX 76102
817-429-1045

Kaplan College—McAllen Campus
1500 S Jackson Rd.
McAllen, TX 78501
956-630-1499

Kaplan College—McAllen Campus
4205 San Pedro Ave.
San Antonio, TX 76212
210-733-0777

Texas State Technical College—Waco
   Campus
3801 Campus Dr.
Waco, TX 76705
817-867-3371

UTAH

American Institute of Medical-Dental
   Technology
1675 N 200 W
Provo, UT 84604
801-377-2900

Provo College
1450 W 820 N
Provo, UT 84601
801-375-1861

Bryman School
1144 W 3300 S
Salt Lake City, UT 84119
801-975-7000

VIRGINIA

Career Development Center
605 Thimble Shoals
Newport News, VA 23606
804-599-4088

Riverside Regional Medical Center—
    School of Professional Nursing
500 J. Clyde Morris Blvd.
Newport News, VA 23601
804-594-2700

National Business College
1813 E Main St.
Salem, VA 24153
540-986-1800

WASHINGTON

Bellingham Technical College
3028 Lindbergh Ave.
Bellingham, WA 98225
360-738-0221

Eton Technical Institute
31919 6th Ave. S
Federal Way, WA 98063
206-941-5800

Lake Washington Technical College
11605 132nd Ave. NE
Kirkland, WA 98034
206-828-5600

Eton Technical Institute
3659 Frontage Rd.
Port Orchard, WA 98366
206-479-3866

Seattle Vocational Institute
315 22nd Ave. S
Seattle, WA 98144
206-587-4950

Spokane Community College
N. 1810 Greene Ave.
Spokane, WA 99207
509-533-7000

Trend College
N 214 Wall St.
Spokane, WA 99201
509-838-3521

Bates Technical College
1101 S Yakima Ave.
Tacoma, WA 98405
206-596-1500

WISCONSIN

Fox Valley Technical College
1825 N Bluemound Dr.
Appleton, WI 54913-2277
414-735-5600

Western Wisconsin Technical College
304 N 6th St., P.O. Box 908
La Crosse, WI 54602-0908
608-785-9200

MEDICAL ASSISTANT TECHNOLOGY

ALABAMA

Gadsden Business College
P.O. Box 1575
Anniston, AL 36202
205-237-7517

New World College of Business
P.O. Box 2287
Anniston, AL 36201
205-236-7578

George C. Wallace State College—Dotham
Rte. 6, P.O. Box 62
Dotham, AL 36303
334-983-3521

Gadsden Business College
750 Forest Ave.
Gadsden, AL 35901
205-546-2863

Capps College
3100 Cottage Hill Rd.
Montgomery, AL 36606
205-473-1393

Coastal Training Institute
5950 Monticello Dr.
Montgomery, AL 36112
205-279-6241

Community College of the Air Force
Maxwell Air Force Base
Montgomery, AL 36112
334-953-6436

ARIZONA

Apollo College—Tri City, Inc.
630 W Southern Ave.
Mesa, AZ 85210
602-831-6585

Institute of Medical and Dental Technology
20 E Main St.
Mesa, AZ 85201
602-969-5505

Apollo College—Phoenix, Inc.
8503 N 27th Ave.
Phoenix, AZ 85051
602-864-1571

Apollo College—Westridge, Inc.
7502 W Thomas Rd.
Phoenix, AZ 85033
602-849-9000

The Bryman School
4343 N 16th St.
Phoenix, AZ 85016
602-274-4300

Gateway Community College
108 N 40th St.
Phoenix, AZ 85034
602-392-5189

The Laural School
2538 N 8th St.
Phoenix, AZ 85006
602-947-6565

Occupational Training Center
4136 N 75th Ave.
Phoenix, AZ 85033
602-849-0308

Apollo College
3870 N Oracle Rd.
Tucson, AZ 85705
520-888-5885

Pima Medical Institute
3350 E Grant Rd.
Tucson, AZ 85710
520-326-1600

ARKANSAS

Eastern College of Health Vocation
6423 Forbing Rd.
Little Rock, AR 72209
501-568-0211

CALIFORNIA

Advanced Computer Training
3467 W Shaw Ave.
Fresno, CA 93703
209-277-1900

American College of Optechs
4021 Rosewood Ave.
Los Angeles, CA 90004
310-383-2862

DISTRICT OF COLUMBIA

Harrison Center for Career Education
624 9th St. NW
Washington, DC 20001
202-628-5672

FLORIDA

William T. McFatter Vocational Technical
  Center
6500 Nova Dr.
Davie, FL 33317
954-370-8324

Keiser College of Technology
1500 NW 49th St.
Fort Lauderdale, FL 33309
305-776-4456

Santa Fe Community College
3000 NW 83rd St.
Gainesville, FL 32601
904-395-5000

Concorde Career Institute
7960 Arlington Expwy.
Jacksonville, FL 32211
904-725-0525

Concorde Career Institute
4000 N State Rd.
Lauderdale Lakes, FL 33319
954-731-8880

Career Training Institute
101 W Main St.
Leesburg, FL 34748
904-326-5134

Phillips Junior College
2401 N Harbor City Blvd.
Melbourne, FL 32935
407-254-6459

Martin Technical College
1901 NW 7th St.
Miami, FL 33125
305-541-8140

Miriam Vocational School, Inc.
7311 W Flagler St.
Miami, FL 33144
305-264-1402

National Education Center—Bauder College
    Campus
7955 NW 12th St.
Miami, FL 33126
305-477-0251

Politechnical Institute of Florida
1405 SW 107th Ave.
Miami, FL 33174
305-226-8099

Miami Lakes Technical Education Center
5780 NW 158th St.
Miami Lakes, FL 33169
305-557-1100

Webster College, Inc.
5623 US Hwy. 19 S
New Port Richey, FL 34652
813-849-4993

Miami Technical College
14701 NW 7th Ave.
North Miami, FL 33168
305-688-8811

National School of Technology, Inc.
16150 NE 17th Ave.
North Miami Beach, FL 33162
305-949-9500

Career Training Institute
2120 W Colonial
Orlando, FL 32804
407-843-3984

Orlando College
5500-5800 Diplomat Cir.
Orlando, FL 32810
407-628-5870

Concorde Career Institute
4202 W Spruce St.
Tampa, FL 33602
813-874-0094

Florida School of Business
4817 Florida Ave. N
Tampa, FL 33603
813-239-3334

Ross Technical Institute
1490 S Military Trail
West Palm Beach, FL 33415
407-433-1288

Tampa College
3319 W Hillsborough Ave.
Tampa, FL 33614
813-879-6000

GEORGIA

Meadows College of Business
832 Slappey Blvd.
Albany, GA 31701
912-883-1736

Athens Area Technical Institute
800 Hwy. 29 N
Athens, GA 30601
706-355-5000

Atlanta Area Technical School
1560 Stewart Ave. SW
Atlanta, GA 30310
404-756-3779

Atlanta College of Medical Dental Careers
1240 W Peachtree St. NE
Atlanta, GA 30309
404-880-8500

Draughons College—Atlanta
1430 Peachtree St.
Atlanta, GA 30309
404-892-0814

National Education Center—Bryman
   Campus
40 Marietta St. NW
Atlanta, GA 30303
404-524-8800

Augusta Technical Institute
3116 Deans Bridge Rd.
Augusta, GA 30906
706-771-4000

Gwinnett Technical Institute
1250 Atkinson Rd., P.O. Box 1505
Lawrenceville, GA 30246
404-962-7580

Medix Schools
2480 Windy Hill Rd.
Marietta, GA 30067
770-980-0002

Savannah Technical Institute
5717 White Bluff Rd.
Savannah, GA 31405-5594
912-352-4362

Thomas Technical Institute
15689 US Hwy. 19 N
Thomasville, GA 31792
912-225-4097

Valdosta Technical Institute
4089 Valtech Rd.
Valdosta, GA 31602
912-333-2100

HAWAII

Medical Assistant School of Hawaii, Inc.
1149 Bethel St.
Honolulu, HI 96813
808-524-3363

IDAHO

American Institute of Health Technology,
   Inc.
1200 N Liberty St.
Boise, ID 83704
208-377-8080

Ricks College
Rexburg, ID 83460
208-356-1020

College of Southern Idaho
P.O. Box 1238
Twin Falls, ID 83301
208-733-9554

ILLINOIS

National Education Center—Bryman

Campus

17 N State Rd.

Chicago, IL 60602

312-368-4911

Robert Morris College

180 N LaSalle St.

Chicago, IL 60601

312-836-4888

INDIANA

Indiana Vocational Technical College—

Southwest

3501 First Ave.

Evansville, IN 47710

812-426-2865

Indiana Vocational Technical College—

North Central

3800 N Anthony Blvd.

Fort Wayne, IN 46805

219-482-9171

International Business College

3811 Illinois Rd.

Fort Wayne, IN 46804

219-432-8702

Professional Career Institute

2611 Waterfront Pkwy., East Dr.

Indianapolis, IN 46214-2028

317-299-6001

Davenport College—Nashville

8200 Georgia St.

Merrillville, IN 46410

219-769-5556

Indiana Vocational Technical College—

South Central

8204 Hwy. 311

Sellersburg, IN 47172

812-246-3301

Michiana College

1030 E Jefferson Blvd.

South Bend, IN 46617

219-237-0774

IOWA

Des Moines Community College

2006 Ankeny Blvd.

Ankeny, IA 50021

515-964-6200

Kirkwood Community College

P.O. Box 2068

Cedar Rapids, IA 52406

319-398-5411

Palmer College of Chiropractic

1000 Brady Dr.

Davenport, IA 52803

800-722-3648

Spencer School of Business

217 W 5th St., P.O. Box 5065

Spencer, IA 51301

712-262-7290

KANSAS

Topeka Technical College

1620 Northwest Gage

Topeka, KS 66618

913-232-5858

Bryan Institute
1004 S Oliver St.
Wichita, KS 67218
316-685-2284

KENTUCKY

Careercom Junior College of Business
1102 S Virginia St.
Hopkinsville, KY 42248
502-886-1302

Kentucky College of Business
628 E Main St.
Lexington, KY 40508
606-253-0621

Spencerian College
4627 Dixie Hwy.
Louisville, KY 40216
502-447-1000

Owensboro Junior College of Business
1515 E 18th St., P.O. Box 1350
Owensboro, KY 42303
502-926-4040

LOUISIANA

Commercial College of Baton Rouge
5677 Florida Blvd.
Baton Rouge, LA 70806
504-927-3470

Domestic Health Care Institute
4826 Jamestown Ave.
Baton Rouge, LA 70808
504-925-5312

Coastal College—Hammond
119 Yokum Rd.
Hammond, LA 70403
504-345-3200

Coastal College—Houma
2318 W Park Ave.
Houma, LA 70364
504-872-2800

Delta Schools, Inc.
4549 Johnston St.
Lafayette, LA 70503
318-988-2211

Southern Technical College
303 Rue Louis XIV
Lafayette, LA 70062
318-981-4010

Eastern College of Health Vocations
3540 I-10 Service Rd. S
Metairie, LA 70001
504-834-8644

Delta Schools, Inc.
413 W Admiral Doyle
New Iberia, LA 70560
318-365-7348

Cameron College
2740 Canal St.
New Orleans, LA 70119
504-821-5881

Coastal College
2001 Canal St.
New Orleans, LA 70119
504-522-2400

National Education Center—Bryman
Campus
2322 Canal St.
New Orleans, LA 70119
504-822-4500

Ayers Institute, Inc.
2924 Knight St.
Shreveport, LA 71105
318-221-1853

Commercial College
2640 Youree Dr.
Shreveport, LA 71104
318-869-4888

Coastal College—Slidell
320 Howze Beach Rd.
Slidell, LA 70481
504-641-2121

MAINE

Mid-State College
88 E Hardscrabble Rd.
Auburn, ME 04210
207-783-1478

Beal College
629 Main St.
Bangor, ME 04401
207-947-4591

Andover College
901 Washington Ave.
Portland, ME 04103
207-774-6126

MARYLAND

Essex Community College
7201 Rossville Blvd.
Baltimore, MD 21237
410-780-6363

Medix Schools
1017 York Rd.
Towson, MD 21204
410-337-5155

MASSACHUSETTS

Bunker Hill Community College
New Rutherford Ave.
Boston, MA 02116
617-228-2027

Fisher College
118 Beacon St.
Boston, MA 02116
617-236-8800

National Education Center—Bryman
Campus
323 Boylston St.
Brookline, MA 02146
617-232-6035

Aquinas College at Newton
15 Walnut Park
Newton, MA 02158
617-969-4400

The Salter School
456 Bridge St.
Springfield, MA 01103
413-731-7353

Associated Technical Institute
345 W Cummings Park
Woburn, MA 01801
617-935-3838

The Salter School
155 Ararat St.
Worcester, MA 01606
508-853-1074

MICHIGAN

Ross Technical Institute
4703 Washtenaw Ave.
Ann Arbor, MI 48108
313-434-7320

Ross Technical Institute
5757 Whitmore Lake Rd.
Brighton, MI 48116
313-227-0160

Ross Business Institute
37065 S Gratiot Ave.
Clinton Township, MI 48036
810-954-3083

Detroit Business Institute
1249 Washington Blvd.
Detroit, MI 48226
313-962-6534

National Education Center—Bryman
   Campus
4244 Oakman Blvd.
Detroit, MI 48204
313-834-1400

Payne-Pullman School of Trade and
   Commerce, Inc.
2345 Cass Ave.
Detroit, MI 48201
313-963-4710

Ross Technical Institute
1553 Woodward Ave.
Detroit, MI 48226
313-965-7451

Ross Medical Education Center
3630 Miller Rd., Ste. D
Flint, MI 48532
810-733-7488

Grand Rapids Educational Center
1750 Woodworth St. NE
Grand Rapids, MI 49505
616-364-8464

Ross Medical Education Center
2035 28th St. SE
Grand Rapids, MI 49508
616-243-3070

Ross Medical Education Center
1188 N West Ave.
Jackson, MI 49202
517-782-7677

Lansing Community College
419 N Capitol Ave.
Lansing, MI 48901
517-483-9850

Ross Medical Education Center
4106 W. Jaginaw Hwy.
Lansing, MI 48917
517-703-9044

National Education Center—National
    Institute of Technology
18000 Newburgh Rd.
Livonia, MI 48152
313-464-7387

Schoolcraft College
18600 Haggerty Rd.
Livonia, MI 48152
313-462-4400

Ross Business Institute
1285 N Telegraph Rd.
Monroe, MI 48161
313-243-5456

Professional Careers Institute
23300 Greenfield Rd.
Oak Park, MI 48237
810-967-2500

Ross Technical Institute
20820 Greenfield Rd.
Oak Park, MI 48237
313-967-3100

Pontiac Business Institute—Oxford
775 W Drahner Rd.
Oxford, MI 48237
313-628-4846

Detroit Business Educational Center
19100 Fort St.
Riverview, MI 48192
313-479-0660

Ross Business Institute
22293 Eureka Rd.
Taylor, MI 48180
313-563-0640

Carnegie Institute
550 Stephenson Hwy.
Troy, MI 48083
810-589-1078

Delta College
1961 Delta Rd.
University Center, MI 48710
517-686-9000

Macomb Community College
14500 Twelve Mile Rd.
Warren, MI 48093
810-445-7999

Ross Medical Education Center
950 Norton Ave., Ste. D
Roosevelt Park, MI 49441
616-739-1531

Ross Medical Education Center
4300 Fashion Square Blvd.
Saginaw, MI 48603
989-791-5792

Ross Medical Education Center
253 Summit Dr.
Pontiac, MI 48053
313-683-1166

National Education Center—National
    Institute of Technology
2620 Remico St. SW
Wyoming, MI 40509
616-538-3170

MINNESOTA

Medical Institute of Minnesota
5503 Green Valley Dr.
Bloomington, MN 55437
612-844-0064

Duluth Business University, Inc.
412 W Superior St.
Duluth, MN 55802
218-722-3361

Northwest Technical College—East Grand
   Forks
Hwy. 220 N
East Grand Forks, MN 56721
218-773-3441

Concorde Career Institute
12 N 12th St.
Minneapolis, MN 55403
612-341-3850

Globe College of Business
175 5th St., P.O. Box 60
Saint Paul, MN 55101
612-224-4378

Lakeland Medical and Dental Academy
1402 W Lake St.
Minneapolis, MN 55408
612-827-5656

Rochester Community College
851 30th Ave. SE
Rochester, MN 55904
507-285-7210

MISSOURI

Bryan Institute
12184 Natural Bridge Rd.
Bridgeton, MO 63044
314-291-0241

Metro Business College of Cape Girardeau
1732 N Kingshighway
Cape Girardeau, MO 63701
314-334-9181

Metro Business College
1407 Southwest Blvd.
Jefferson City, MO 65109
314-635-6600

Concorde Career Institute
3239 Broadway
Kansas City, MO 64111
816-531-5223

Tad Technical Institute
7910 Troost Ave.
Kansas City, MO 64131
816-361-5640

Midwest Institute for Medical Assistants
112 W Jefferson Ave.
Kirkwood, MO 63122
314-965-8363

Metro Business College
1202 E Hwy. 72
Rolla, MO 65401
314-364-8464

Al-Med Academy
10963 Saint Charles Rock Rd.
Saint Louis, MO 63074
314-739-4450

Missouri School for Doctors' Assistants
10121 Manchester Rd.
Saint Louis, MO 63122
314-821-7700

Saint Louis College of Health Careers
909 S Taylor Ave.
Saint Louis, MO 63108
314-652-0300

Phillips Junior College
1010 W Sunshine St.
Springfield, MO 65807
417-864-7220

NEBRASKA

Southeast Community College—Lincoln
    Campus
8800 O St.
Lincoln, NE 68520
402-471-3333

Institute of Computer Science
808 S 74th Pl., 7400 Court Bldg.
Omaha, NE 68114
402-393-7064

Omaha College of Health Careers
10845 Harney St.
Omaha, NE 68154
402-333-1400

NEVADA

American Academy for Career
    Education
3120 E Desert Inn Rd.
Las Vegas, NV 89121
702-732-7748

Canterbury Career Schools
2215C Renaissance Dr.
Las Vegas, NV 89119
702-798-6929

NEW HAMPSHIRE

New Hampshire Technical College at
    Claremont
1 College Dr.
Claremont, NH 03743
603-542-7744

NEW JERSEY

Omega Institute
Rte. 130 S Cinnaminson Mall
Cinnaminson, NJ 08077
609-786-2200

Star Technical Institute—Deptford
251 Delsea Dr.
Deptford, NJ 08104
609-384-2888

Dover Business College
15 E Blackwell St.
Dover, NJ 07801
201-366-6700

Barclay Career School
28 S Harrison St.
E Orange, NJ 07017
201-673-0500

Star Technical Institute
2224 US Hwy. 130, Park Plaza
Edgewater Park, NJ 08010
609-877-2727

Drake College of Business
9 Caldwell Pl.
Elizabeth, NJ 07201
201-352-5509

American Business Academy
66 Moore St.
Hackensack, NJ 07601
201-488-9400

Star Technical Institute
1255 Rte. 70
Lakewood, NJ 08701
908-901-9710

Star Technical Institute—Oakhurst
2105 Hwy. 35
Oakhurst, NJ 07755
908-493-1660

Business Training Institute
4 Forest Ave.
Paramus, NJ 07652
201-845-9300

Ho-Ho-Kus School
27 S Franklin Tpke.
Ramsey, NJ 07446
201-327-8877

Berdan Institute
265 Rte. 46
Totowa, NJ 07512
201-256-3444

NEW MEXICO

Franklin Medical College—Branch Campus
2400 Louisiana Blvd. NE
Albuquerque, NM 87110
505-883-4800

Pima Medical Institute
2201 San Pedro Dr. NE
Albuquerque, NM 87110
505-881-1234

NEW YORK

Bryant and Stratton Business Institute—
    Buffalo
1028 Main St.
Buffalo, NY 14202
716-884-9120

Suburban Technical School
2650 Sunrise Hwy.
East Islip, NY 11730
516-224-5001

New York School for Medical and Dental
    Assistants
116-16 Queens Blvd.
Forest Hills, NY 11375
718-793-2330

Suburban Technical School
175 Fulton Ave.
Hempstead, NY 11550
516-481-6660

Blake Business School—New York City
20 Cooper Sq.
New York, NY 10003
212-254-1233

Mandl School
254 W 54th St.
New York, NY 10019
212-247-3434

Hudson Valley Community College
80 Vandenburgh Ave.
Troy, NY 12180
518-283-1100

NORTH CAROLINA

Central Piedmont Community College
P.O. Box 35009
Charlotte, NC 28235
704-342-6633

Pitt Community College
P.O. Drawer 7007
Greenville, NC 27835
919-321-4200

Miller-Motte Business College
606 S College Rd.
Wilmington, NC 28403
910-392-4660

NORTH DAKOTA

Interstate Business College
520 E Main Ave.
Bismarck, ND 58501
701-255-0779

Interstate Business College
2720 32nd Ave. SW
Fargo, ND 58103
701-232-2477

OHIO

Akron Medical-Dental Institute
733 W Marker St.
Akron, OH 44303
216-762-9788

Mahoning County Joint Vocational School
    District
7300 N Palmyra Rd.
Canfield, OH 44406
216-533-3923

Fairfield Career Center
4000 Columbus Lancaster Rd.
Carroll, OH 43112
614-836-4541

RETS Technical Center
116 Westpark Rd.
Centerville, OH 45459
513-433-3410

Institute of Medical-Dental Technology
4452 Eastgate Blvd.
Cincinnati, OH 45246
513-753-5030

Institute of Medical-Dental Technology
375 Glensprings Dr.
Cincinnati, OH 45246
513-851-8500

Cleveland Institute of Dental-Medical
   Assistants
1836 Euclid Ave.
Cleveland, OH 44115
216-241-2930

Cuyahoga Community College District
700 Carnegie Ave.
Cleveland, OH 44115
216-987-6000

MTI Business College
1140 Euclid Ave
Cleveland, OH 44115
216-621-8228

National Education Center
14445 Broadway Ave.
Cleveland, OH 44125
216-475-7520

Sawyer College of Business
3150 Mayfield Rd.
Cleveland Heights, OH 44118
216-932-0911

American School of Technology
2100 Morse Rd.
Columbus, OH 43229
614-436-4820

Columbus Para Professional Institute
1077 Lexington Ave.
Columbus, OH 43201
614-299-0200

Technology Education Center
288 S Hamilton Rd.
Columbus, OH 43213
614-759-7700

National Education Center—National
   Institute of Technology
1225 Orlen Ave.
Cuyahoga Falls, OH 44221
216-923-9959

Southwestern College of Business
225 W 1st St.
Dayton, OH 48402
513-294-2103

Warren County Career Center
3525 N SR 48
Lebanon, OH 45036
513-932-5677

ESI Career Center
1985 N Ridge Rd. E
Lorain, OH 44055
216-277-8832

Cleveland Institute of Dental-Medical
   Assistants
5733 Hopkins Rd.
Mentor, OH 44060
216-946-9530

Knox County Career Center
306 Martinsburg Rd.
Mount Vernon, OH 43050
614-397-5820

Tri-County Vocational School
15675 SR 691
Nelsonville, OH 45764
614-753-3511

Boheckers Business College
326 E Main St.
Ravenna, OH 44266
330-297-7319

Belmont Technical College
120 Fox Shannon Pl.
Saint Clairsville, OH 43950
614-695-9500

Professional Skills Institute
5115 Glendale Ave.
Toledo, OH 43614
419-720-6670

Stautzenberger College
5355 Southwyck Blvd.
Toledo, OH 43614
419-866-5167

University of Toledo
2801 W Bancroft St.
Toledo, OH 43606
419-537-2072

Trumbull County Joint Vocational School
   District
528 Educational Hwy.
Warren, OH 44483
216-847-0503

OKLAHOMA

Southern Oklahoma Area Vocational-
   Technical Center
2610 Sam Noble Pky.
Ardmore, OK 73401
405-223-2070

Platt College
6125 W Reno Ave.
Oklahoma City, OK 73127
405-789-5052

De Marge College
3608 NW 58th St.
Oklahoma City, OK 73112
405-947-1425

Francis Tuttle Area Vocational-Technical
   Center
12777 N Rockwell Ave.
Oklahoma City, OK 73142-2789
405-722-7799

Wright Business School
2219 SW 74th St.
Oklahoma City, OK 73159
405-681-2300

Central Technology Center
1720 S Main St.
Sapulpa, OK 74030
918-224-9300

Bryan Institute
2843 E 51st St.
Tulsa, OK 74105
918-749-6891

OREGON

Apollo College-Portland, Inc.
2600 SE 98th Ave.
Portland, OR 97266
503-761-6100

College of America
921 SW Washington St.
Portland, OR 97205
503-242-9000

Western Business College
425 SW 6th Ave.
Portland, OR 97204
503-222-3225

Pioneer Pacific College
25195 SW Parkway Ave.
Wilsonville, OR 97070
503-682-3903

PENNSYLVANIA

Altoona Area Vocational Technology School
1500 4th Ave.
Altoona, PA 16602
814-946-8490

Allied Medical Centers, Inc.
104 Woodward Rd.
Edwardsville, PA 18704
717-288-8400

J. H. Thompson Academies
2910 State Rd.
Erie, PA 16508
814-456-6217

Academy of Medical Arts and Business
279 Boas St.
Harrisburg, PA 17102
717-233-2172

National Education Center—Thompson
   Institute Campus
5650 Derry St.
Harrisburg, PA 17111
717-564-4112

Star Technical Institute—Kingston
212 Wyoming Ave.
Kingston, PA 18704
717-829-6960

Career Training Academy
244 Center Rd.
Monroeville, PA 15146
412-372-3900

Career Training Academy
703 5th Ave.
New Kensington, PA 15068
412-337-1000

The Craft Institute
27 S 12th St.
Philadelphia, PA 19107
215-592-4600

Delaware Valley Academy of Medical and
   Dental Assistants
3330 Grant Ave.
Philadelphia, PA 19114
215-676-1200

National Education Center
3440 Marker St.
Philadelphia, PA 19104
215-387-1530

Duffs Business Institute
110 9th St.
Pittsburgh, PA 15222
412-261-4520

ICM School of Business
10-14 Wood St.
Pittsburgh, PA 15222
412-261-2647

Median School of Allied Health Careers
125 7th St.
Pittsburgh, PA 15222-3400
800-570-0693

North Hills School of Health Occupations
1500 Northway Mall
Pittsburgh, PA 15237
412-367-8003

Sawyer School
717 Liberty Ave.
Pittsburgh, PA 15222
412-261-5700

Antonelli Medical and Professional Institute
1700 Industrial Pkwy.
Pottstown, PA 19464
610-323-7270

Allied Medical Careers, Inc.
2901 Pittston Ave.
Scranton, PA 18505
717-342-8000

Star Technical Institute—Whitehall
1541 Alta Dr.
Whitehall, PA 18052
215-434-9963

Berks Technical Institute
832 N Park Rd., 4 Park Plaza
Wyomissing, PA 19610
215-372-1722

SOUTH CAROLINA
Trident Technical College
P.O. Box 118067
Charleston, SC 29423-8067
803-572-6111

Central Carolina Technical College
506 N Guignard Dr.
Sumter, SC 29150
803-778-1961

TENNESSEE
Draughon College
3200 Elvis Presley Blvd.
Memphis, TN 38116
901-332-7800

Davidson Technical College
212 Pavillion Blvd.
Nashville, TN 37217
615-360-3300

Fugazzi College
5042 Linbar Dr.
Nashville, TN 37217
615-333-3344

Medical Career College
537 Main St.
Nashville, TN 37206
901-644-7365

TEXAS

Bryan Institute
1719 Pioneer Pkwy. W
Arlington, TX 76013
817-265-5588

Southern Careers Institute
2301 S Congress Ave.
Austin, TX 78704
512-326-1415

ATI Health Education Center
8150 Brookriver Dr.
Dallas, TX 75247
214-637-0980

PCI Health Training Center
8101 John Carpenter Fwy.
Dallas, TX 75247
214-263-8724

Career Centers of Texas El Paso, Inc.
8375 Brunham Dr.
El Paso, TX 79907
915-595-1935

Western Technical Institute
4710 Alabama St., P.O. Box M
El Paso, TX 79951
915-566-9621

ATI Health Education Center
1200 Summit Ave.
Fort Worth, TX 76102
817-429-1045

Avalon Vocational Technical Institute
1407 Texas St.
Fort Worth, TX 76102
817-877-5511

The Academy of Health Care Professions
1919 N Loop W
Houston, TX 77008
713-741-2633

Bradford School of Business
4669 Southwest Hwy.
Houston, TX 77027
713-629-8940

National Education Center—Bryman
  Campus
9724 Beechnut, Ste. 300
Houston, TX 77036

National Education Center—Bryman
  Campus
16416 N Chase Dr.
Houston, TX 77060

Southern Careers Institute—South Texas
3233 N 38th St.
McAllen, TX 78501
210-687-1415

Avalon Vocational Technical Institute
4241 Tanglewood Ln.
Odessa, TX 79762
915-367-2622

Southwest School of Business and
  Technical Careers
3900 N 23rd
McAllen, TX 78501
956-687-7007

National Education Center—NIT Campus
3622 Fredericksburg Rd.
San Antonio, TX 78201
210-733-6000

San Antonio College of Medical and Dental
   Assistants—Central
4205 San Pedro Ave.
San Antonio, TX 78212
210-733-0777

San Antonio College of Medical and Dental
   Assistants
5280 Medical Dr.
San Antonio, TX 78229
210-692-0241

Southwest School of Business and
   Technical Careers
602 W South Cross
San Antonio, TX 78221
512-921-0951

Southwest School of Medical Assistants
201 W Sheridan
San Antonio, TX 78204
512-224-2296

UTAH

Stevens-Henager College of Business
2168 Washington Blvd.
Ogden, UT 84401
801-394-7791

American Institute of Medical-Dental
   Technology
1675 N 200 W
Provo, UT 84604
801-377-2900

Stevens-Henager College of Business
25 E 1700 S
Provo, UT 84606
801-375-5455

Bryman School
1144 W 3300 S
Salt Lake City, UT 84119
801-975-7000

VIRGINIA

Career Development Center
605 Thimble Shoals
Newport News, VA 23606
804-599-4088

Commonwealth College
300 Boush St.
Norfolk, VA 23510
804-625-5891

National Education Center—Kee Business
   College Campus
861 Glenrock Rd.
Norfolk, VA 23418
804-461-2922

Tidewater Technical
1760 E Little Creek Rd.
Norfolk, VA 23518
804-588-2121

National Education Center—Kee Business
   College Campus
6301 Midlothian Tpke.
Richmond, VA 23225
804-745-3300

Dominion Business School
4142-1 Melrose Ave.
Roanoke, VA 24017
703-362-7738

Commonwealth College
4160 Virginia Beach Blvd.
Virginia Beach, VA 23452
804-340-0222

Tidewater Technical
2697 Dean Dr.
Virginia Beach, VA 23452
804-340-2121

WASHINGTON

Eton Technical Institute
209 E Casino Rd.
Everett, WA 98204
206-353-4888

Eton Technical Institute
31919 6th Ave. S
Federal Way, WA 98063
206-941-5800

Eton Technical Institute
3649 Frontage Rd.
Port Orchard, WA 98366
206-479-3866

Pima Medical Institute
1627 Eastlake Ave. E
Seattle, WA 98102
206-322-6100

Seattle Vocational Institute
315 22nd Ave. S
Seattle, WA 98144
206-587-4950

Spokane Community College
N 1810 Greene Ave.
Spokane, WA 99201
509-536-7000

Trend College
N 214 Wall St.
Spokane, WA 99201
509-838-3521

WEST VIRGINIA

Boone County Career & Technical Center
P.O. Box 50B
Danville, WV 25053
304-369-4585

Huntington Junior College
900 5th Ave.
Huntington, WV 25701
304-697-7550

Opportunities Industrialization Center—
    North Central West Virginia
120 Jackson St.
Fairmont, WV 26554
304-366-8142

West Virginia Career College
148 Willey St.
Morgantown, WV 26505
304-296-8282

WISCONSIN

Northeast Wisconsin Technical College
2740 W Mason St., P.O. Box 19042
Green Bay, WI 54307-9042
414-498-5400

Blackhawk Technical College
P.O. Box 5009
Janesville, WI 53547
608-756-4121

Madison Area Technical College
3550 Anderson St.
Madison, WI 53704
608-246-6100

Milwaukee Area Technical College
700 W State St.
Milwaukee, WI 53233
414-297-6600

Waukesha County Technical College
800 Main St.
Pewaukee, WI 53072
414-691-5566

Wisconsin Indianhead Technical College
505 Pine Ridge Dr., P.O. Box 10B
Shell Lake, WI 54871
715-468-2815

Mid-State Technical College—Main Campus
500 32nd St. N
Wisconsin Rapids, WI 54494
715-423-5650

NURSING ASSISTANT TECHNOLOGY

ALABAMA

Read State Technical College
P.O. Box 588
Evergreen, AL 36401
205-578-1313

Trenholm State Technical College
1225 Air Base Blvd.
Montgomery, AL 36108
334-832-9000

Bevill State Community College
P.O. Box Drawer K
Sumiton, AL 35148
205-648-3271

ARIZONA

Gateway Community College
108 N 40th St.
Phoenix, AZ 80534
602-392-5000

Eastern Arizona College
600 Church St.
Thatcher, AZ 85552
602-428-8322

Pima Community College
2202 W Anklam Rd.
Tucson, AZ 85709
520-206-6640

Pima Medical College
3350 Grant Rd.
Tucson, AZ 85716
520-326-1600

Tucson College
7302-10 E 22nd St.
Tucson, AZ 85710
520-296-3261

ARKANSAS

Gateway Technical College
P.O. Box 3350
Batesville, AR 72503
501-793-7581

Crowley's Ridge Technical School
P.O. Box 925
Forrest City, AR 72335
501-633-5411

Eastern College of Health Vocation
6423 Forbing Rd.
Little Rock, AR 72209
501-568-0211

Great Rivers Vocational-Technical School
P.O. Box 747
McGehee, AR 71654
501-222-5360

Arkansas Valley Technical Institute
Hwy. 23 N, P.O. Box 4506
Ozark, AR 72949
501-667-2117

Black River Technical College
Hwy. 304, P.O. Box 468
Pocahontas, AR 72455
501-892-4565

CALIFORNIA

American School of X-Ray
13723 Harvard Pl.
Gardena, CA 90249
213-770-4001

Hacienda La Puente Unified School
　　　District—Valley Vocational Center
15959 E Gale Ave.
La Puente, CA 91749
818-968-4638

Educorp Career College
230 E 3rd St.
Long Beach, CA 90802
213-437-0501

Allied Nursing Center, Inc.
3806 Beverly Blvd.
Los Angeles, CA 90064
213-389-9337

Nova Institute of Health Technology
520 N Euclid Ave.
Ontario, CA 91762
909-984-5027

Butte College
3536 Butte Campus Dr.
Oroville, CA 95965
916-895-2511

Mission College
3000 Mission College Blvd.
Santa Clara, CA 95054
408-748-2700

Allan Hancock College
800 S College Dr.
Santa Maria, CA 93454
805-922-6966

Santa Rosa Junior College
1501 Mendocino Ave.
Santa Rosa, CA 95401
707-527-4100

Simi Valley Adult School
3192 Los Angeles Ave.
Simi Valley, CA 93065
805-527-4840

COLORADO

San Luis Valley Area Vocational School
1011 Main St.
Alamosa, CO 81101
719-589-5871

Colorado Mountain College
P.O. Box 10001
Glenwood Springs, CO 81620
970-945-7481

PPI Health Careers School
2345 N Academy Blvd.
Colorado Springs, CO 80909
719-596-7400

CONNECTICUT

Connecticut Business Institute
809 Main St.
East Hartford, CT 06108
203-291-2880

Conecticut Business Institute
605 Broad St.
Stratford, CT 06497
203-377-1775

FLORIDA

Atlantic Vocational Technical Center
4700 Coconut Creek Pkwy.
Coconut Creek, FL 33063
954-977-2000

Brevard Community College
1519 Clearlake Rd.
Fort Lauderdale, FL 33304
407-632-1111

Beacon Career Institute, Inc.
2900 NW 183rd St.
Miami, FL 33056
305-620-4637

Nurse Assistant Training School, Inc.
5154 Okeechobee Blvd.
West Palm Beach, FL 33417
561-683-1400

MASSACHUSETTS

Assabet Valley Regional Vocational
   Technical School
215 Fitchburg St.
Marlborough, MA 01752
508-485-9430

MICHIGAN

Ross Medical Education Center
3630 Miller Rd., Ste. D
Flint, MI 48532
810-230-1100

Detroit Business Institute
1249 Washington Blvd.
Detroit, MI 48226
313-962-6534

Ross Technical Institute
1553 Woodward
Detroit, MI 48226
313-371-2131

Ross Medical Education Center
15670 E Eight Mile Rd.
Detroit, MI 48205

Ross Technical Institute
20820 Greenfield Rd.
Oak Park, MI 48237
313-967-3100

Ross Medical Education Center
950 Norton Ave., Ste. D
Roosevelt Park, MI 49441
616-739-1531

Ross Medical Education Center
4300 Fashion Square Blvd.
Saginaw, MI 46803
989-791-5792

MINNESOTA

Duluth Technical College
2101 Trinity Rd.
Duluth, MN 55811
218-722-2801

Itasca Community College
1851 Hwy. 169 E
Grand Rapids, MN 55744
218-327-4460

Northeast Metro Technical College
3300 Century Ave. N
White Bear Lake, MN 55110
612-770-2351

MISSISSIPPI

Northwest Mississippi Community College
Hwy. 51 N
Senatobia, MS 38668
601-562-5262

MISSOURI

Cape Girardeau Area Vocational-Technical
   School
301 N Clarke Ave.
Cape Girardeau, MO 63701
314-334-3358

Saint Louis College of Health Careers
4484 W Pine Blvd.
Saint Louis, MO 63108
314-652-0300

Sikeston Area Vocational Technical School
1002 Virginia St.
Sikeston, MO 63801
314-472-2581

MONTANA

Dawson Community College
300 College Dr.
Glendive, MT 59330
406-365-3396

Great Falls Vocational Technical Center
2100 16th Ave. S
Great Falls, MT 59405
406-791-2100

NEBRASKA

Opportunity Industrialization Center Omaha
2724 N 24th St.
Omaha, NE 68111
402-457-4222

NEW MEXICO

Albuquerque Technical-Vocational Institute
525 Buena Vista SE
Albuquerque, NM 87106
505-224-3000

Franklin Medical College—Branch Campus
2400 Louisiana Blvd. NE
Albuquerque, NM 87110
505-883-4800

Crownpoint Institute of Technology
P.O. Box 849
Crownpoint, NM 87313
505-786-5851

NEW YORK

CM First Step Training Center
1360 Fulton St.
Brooklyn, NY 11242
718-783-5656

Municipal Training Center
44 Court St.
Brooklyn, NY 11201
718-855-4144

A Business Career Institute, Inc.
91-31 Queens Blvd.
Elmhurst, NY 11373
718-458-1500

Suburban Technical School
175 Fulton Ave.
Hempstead, NY 11550
516-481-6660

Cashier Training Institute
500 8th Ave.
New York, NY 10018
212-564-0500

New York Training Institute for NLP
145 Ave. of the Americas
New York, NY 10012
212-647-1600

Superior Career Institute, Inc.
116 W 14th St.
New York, NY 10038
212-675-2140

Travel Institute
15 Park Row
New York, NY 10038
212-349-3331

NORTH CAROLINA

Roanoke-Chowan Community College
Rte. 2, P.O. Box 46A
Ahoeskie, NC 27910
919-332-5921

Coastal Carolina Community College
444 Western Blvd.
Jacksonville, NC 28546-6877
910-938-6246

Robeson Community College
P.O. Box 1420
Lumberton, NC 28359
910-738-7101

Craven Community College
800 College Ct.
New Bern, NC 28562
919-638-4131

Piedmont Community College
P.O. Box 1197
Roxboro, NC 27573
910-599-1181

Brunswick Community College
P.O. Box 30
Supply, NC 28461
910-754-6900

NORTH DAKOTA

Meyer Vocational Technical School
2045 NW 3rd, P.O. Box 2126
Minot, ND 58702
701-852-0427

OHIO

Madison Local Schools—Madison Adult
   Education
600 Esley Ln.
Mansfield, OH 44905
419-589-6363

Tri-Rivers Career Center
2222 Marion Mount Gilead Rd.
Marion, OH 43302
614-389-6347

Gallia Jackson Vinton JUSD
P.O. Box 157
Rio Grande, OH 45674
614-245-5334

OKLAHOMA

Southwest Area Vocational-Technical
   Center
1121 N Spurgeon St.
Altus, OK 73521
405-477-2250

Mid-Del College
3420 S Sunnylane Rd.
Del City, OK 73115
405-677-8311

Tulsa County Area Vocational-Technological
   School District 18
3802 N Peoria Ave.
Tulsa, OK 74106
918-428-2261

OREGON

Southwestern Oregon Community College
1988 Newmark Ave.
Coos Bay, OR 97420
541-888-7339

PENNSYLVANIA

Delaware County Institute of Training
615 Ave. of the States
Chester, PA 19013
610-874-1888

Allied Medical Careers, Inc.
104 Woodward Hill Rd.
Edwardsville, PA 18704
717-288-8400

Pennsylvania State University—Allentown
    Campus
6090 Mohr Ln.
Fogelsville, PA 18051-9733
610-821-6577

McKeesport Hospital School of Nursing
    Assistants
1500 5th Ave.
McKeesport, PA 15132
412-664-2139

American Institute of Design
1616 Orthodox St.
Philadelphia, PA 19124
215-288-8200

Antonelli Medical and Professional Institute
1700 Industrial Hwy.
Pottstown, PA 19664
610-323-7270

Presbyterian Home Nurse Assistant School
P.O. Box 551
Phillipsburg, PA 16866
814-342-6090

Allied Medical Careers, Inc.
2901 Pittston Ave.
Scranton, PA 18505
717-288-8400

Advanced Career Training
SW Corner 69th & Markey
Upper Darby, PA 19505
610-352-3600

SOUTH CAROLINA

Chris Logan Career College
1125 15-401 Bypass
Bennettsville, SC 29512
803-479-4076

Chris Logan Career College
P.O. Box 261
Myrtle Beach, SC 29578
803-448-6302

Chris Logan Career College
256 S Pike Rd.
Sumter, SC 29150
803-775-2667

Trident Technical College
P.O. Box 118067
Charleston, SC 29423
803-572-6215

TENNESSEE

Elizabethton State Area Vocational
Technical School
1500 Arney St., P.O. Box 789
Elizabethton, TN 37643
615-542-4174

Tennessee Technology Center at
Hohenwald
813 W Main St.
Hohenwald, TN 38462
931-796-5351

Knoxville State Area Vocational-Technical
School
1100 Liberty St.
Knoxville, TN 37919
423-546-5568

Rice College
1515 Magnolia Ave. NE
Knoxville, TN 37917
423-637-9899

Draughons College
3200 Elvis Presley Blvd.
Memphis, TN 38116
901-332-7800

Memphis Area Vocational-Technical School
550 Alabama Ave.
Memphis, TN 38105
901-543-6100

Rice College
1399 Madison Ave.
Memphis, TN 38104
901-725-1000

Davidson Technical College
212 Pavilion Blvd.
Nashville, TN 37217
615-360-3300

Medical Career College
537 Main St.
Nashville, TN 37206
615-255-7531

Paris State Area Vocational-Technical
School
312 S Wilson St.
Paris, TN 38242
901-644-7365

TEXAS

Delta Career Institute
1310 Pennsylvania Ave.
Beaumont, TX 77701
409-833-6161

Brazos Business College
1702 S Texas Ave.
Bryan, TX 77802
409-822-6423

Southwest School of Business and
Technical Careers
272 Commercial St.
Eagle Pass, TX 78852
512-773-1373

Texas State Technical College—Harlingen
Campus
1902 N Loop
Harlingen, TX 78550
956-364-4000

Houston Medical Career Training, Inc.
2420 Garland Dr.
Houston, TX 77087
713-641-6300

Transworld Academy, Inc.
6220 Westpark Dr.
Houston, TX 77057
713-266-6594

Southern Careers Institute—South Texas
3233 N 38th St.
McAllen, TX 78501
956-687-1415

Chenier
2819 Loop 306
San Angelo, TX 76904
915-944-4404

Southwest School of Business and
  Technical Careers
602 W Southcross Blvd.
San Antonio, TX 78221
210-921-0951

UTAH

Bridgerland Applied Technology Center
1301 N 600 W
Logan, UT 84321
801-753-6780

Salt Lake Community College—Skills
  Center
South City Campus, 1575 S State St.
Salt Lake City, UT 84115
801-957-3354

VIRGINIA

Southside Training Skill Center Nottoway
  County
P.O. Box 258
Crewe, VA 23930
804-645-7471

Career Development Center
605 Thimble Shoals
Newport News, VA 23606
804-599-4088

Tidewater Technical
616 Denbigh Blvd.
Newport News, VA 23602
804-874-2121

Tidewater Technical
1760 E Little Creek Rd.
Norfolk, VA 23518
804-588-2121

Blue Ridge Nursing Home School
Commerce St., P.O. Box 459
Stuart, VA 24171
703-694-7161

Tidewater Technical
2697 Dean Dr.
Virginia Beach, VA 23452
804-340-2121

WASHINGTON

Lower Columbia College
P.O. Box 3010
Longview, WA 98632
206-577-2300

Big Bend Community College
7662 Chanute St. NE
Moses Lake, WA 98837
509-793-2222

Bates Technical College
1101 S Yakima Ave.
Tacoma, WA 98405
206-596-1500

Yakima Valley Community College
P.O. Box 1647
Yakima, WA 98907
509-574-4712

WISCONSIN

Fox Valley Technical College
1825 N Bluemound Dr.
Appleton, WI 54913
414-735-5600

Lakeshore Vocational Training and Adult
    Education System District
1290 North Ave.
Cleveland, WI 53015
414-458-4183

Southwest Wisconsin Technical College
Hwy. 18 E
Fennimore, WI 53809
608-822-3262

Wisconsin Area Vocational Training and
    Adult Education System—Moraine Park
235 N National Ave., P.O. Box 1940
Fond du Lac, WI 54936
414-922-8611

Northwest Wisconsin Technical College
2740 W Mason St., P.O. Box 19042
Green Bay, WI 54307
414-498-5400

Blackhawk Technical College
P.O. Box 5009
Janesville, WI 53547
608-756-4121

Gateway Technical College
3520 30th Ave.
Kenosha, WI 53144
414-656-6900

Western Wisconsin Technical College
304 N 6th St., P.O. Box 908
La Crosse, WI 54602
608-785-9200

Madison Area Technical College
3550 Anderson St.
Madison, WI 53704
608-246-6100

Milwaukee Area Technical College
700 W State St.
Milwaukee, WI 53233
414-297-6600

Waukesha County Technical College
800 Main St.
Pewaukee, WI 53072
414-691-5566

Nicolet Vocational Training and Adult Educa-
    tion System District
P.O. Box 518
Rhinelander, WI 54501
715-365-4410

Wisconsin Indianhead Technical College
505 Pine Ridge Dr., P.O. Box 108
Shell Lake, WI 54871
715-468-2815

North Central Technical College
1000 Campus Dr.
Wausau, WI 54401
715-675-3331

Mid-State Technical College—Main Campus
500 32nd St. N
Wisconsin Rapids, WI 54494
715-423-5650

PHYSICAL THERAPY ASSISTANT TECHNOLOGY

ALABAMA

University of Alabama at Birmingham
UAB MJH 107 2010
Birmingham, AL 35294
205-934-3443

George C. Wallace State Community
    College—Hanceville
801 Main St. NW, P.O. Box 2000
Hanceville, AL 35077
205-352-6403

Community College of the Air Force
Maxwell Air Force Base
Montgomery, AL 36112
334-953-6436

ARIZONA

Long Medical Institute
4126 N Black Canyon Hwy.
Phoenix, AZ 85017
602-279-9333

Pima Medical Institute
2300 E Broadway Rd.
Tempe, AZ 85282
602-345-7777

ARKANSAS

University of Central Arkansas
201 Donaghey Ave.
Conway, AR 72035
501-450-5000

CALIFORNIA

De Anza College
21250 Stevens Creek Blvd.
Cupertino, CA 95014
408-864-5678

Imperial Valley College
P.O. Box 158
Imperial, CA 92251
619-352-8320

Loma Linda University
Loma Linda, CA 92350
909-824-4931

Cerritos College
11110 Alondra Blvd.
Norwalk, CA 90650
310-860-2451

Sawyer College at Ventura
2101 E Gonzales Rd.
Oxnard, CA 93030
805-485-6000

COLORADO
Aims Community College
P.O. Box 69
Greeley, CO 80632
970-330-8008

CONNECTICUT
Manchester Community College
60 Bidwell St., P.O. Box 1045
Manchester, CT 06040
203-647-6000

FLORIDA
Broward Community College
225 E Las Olas Blvd.
Fort Lauderdale, FL 33301
954-761-7464

Miami-Dade Community College
300 NE 2nd Ave.
Miami, FL 33132
305-237-3336

Charlotte Vocational-Technical Center
18300 Toledo Blade Blvd.
Port Charlotte, FL 33948
941-629-6819

Saint Petersburg Junior College
P.O. Box 13489
Saint Petersburg, FL 33733
813-341-3611

GEORGIA
Athens Area Technical Institute
800 Hwy. 29 N
Athens, GA 30601
706-542-8050

Gwinnett Technical Institute
1250 Atkinson Rd., P.O. Box 1505
Lawrenceville, GA 30246
404-962-7580

IDAHO
American Institute of Health Technology, Inc.
1200 N Liberty St.
Boise, ID 83704
208-377-8080

ILLINOIS
Belleville Area College
2500 Carlyle Rd.
Belleville, IL 62221
618-235-2700

Morton College
3801 S Central Ave.
Cicero, IL 60650
708-656-8000

KANSAS

Neosho County Community College
800 W 14th St.
Chanute, KS 66720
620-431-6222

Colby Community College
1255 S Range Ave.
Colby, KS 67701
785-462-3984

Cloud County Community College
2221 Campus Dr., P.O. Box 1002
Concordia, KS 66901
913-243-1435

Allen County Community College
1801 N Cottonwood St.
Iola, KS 66749
316-365-5116

Kansas City Area Vocational Technical
 School
2220 N 59th St.
Kansas City, KS 66104
913-596-5500

Kaw Area Vocational-Technical School
5724 SW Huntoon St.
Topeka, KS 66604
913-273-7140

North Central Kansas Area Vocational
 Technical School
P.O. Box 507
Beloit, KS 67420
913-738-2276

Salina Area Vocational Technical School
2562 Scanlan Ave.
Salina, KS 67401
913-825-2261

Wichita Area Technical College
301 S Grove St.
Wichita, KS 67211
316-677-9400

MARYLAND

Baltimore City Community College
2901 Liberty Heights Ave.
Baltimore, MD 21215
410-333-5555

MASSACHUSETTS

Newbury College
129 Fisher Ave.
Brookline, MA 02146
617-730-7000

Becker College—Worcester
61 Sever St.
Worcester, MA 01615
508-791-9241

MICHIGAN

Delta College
1961 Delta Rd.
University Center, MI 48710
517-686-9093

Macomb Community College
14500 Twelve Mile Rd.
Warren, MI 48093
810-445-7000

MINNESOTA

Anoka-Ramsey Community College
11200 Mississippi Blvd.
Coon Rapids, MN 55433
612-427-2600

College of Saint Catherine—Saint Mary's
    Campus
2500 S 6th St.
Minneapolis, MN 55454
612-690-7700

MISSOURI

Jefferson College
1000 Viking Dr.
Hillsboro, MO 63050
314-789-3951

NEW JERSEY

University of Medicine and Dentistry of
    New Jersey
65 Bergen St.
Newark, NJ 07107
201-982-4821

NEW YORK

Genesee Community College
1 College Rd.
Batavia, NY 14020
716-343-0055

CUNY Kingsborough Community College
2001 Oriental Blvd.
Brooklyn, NY 11235
718-368-5000

Nassau Community College
1 Education Dr.
Garden City, NY 11530
516-572-7345

CUNY La Guardia Community College
31-10 Thomson Ave.
Long Island City, NY 11101
718-482-7200

Suffolk County Community College—
    Ammerman Campus
533 College Rd.
Selden, NY 11784
516-451-4110

NORTH CAROLINA

Central Piedmont Community College
P.O. Box 35009
Charlotte, NC 28235
704-342-6633

OHIO

Cuyahoga Community College District
700 Carnegie Ave.
Cleveland, OH 44115-2878
216-987-6000

Stark Technical College
6200 Frank Ave. NW
Canton, OH 44720
216-494-6170

Kent State University—East Liverpool
    Regional Campus
400 E 4th St.
East Liverpool, OH 43920
216-385-3805

OREGON

Mount Hood Community College

26000 SE Stark St.

Gresham, OR 97030

513-667-6422

PENNSYLVANIA

Harcom Junior College

Morris and Montgomery Ave.

Bryn Mawr, PA 19010

610-526-6086

Pennsylvania State University—

Hazleton Campus

76 University Dr.

Hazleton, PA 19202

570-450-3000

Community College of Allegheny County

800 Allegheny Ave.

Pittsburgh, PA 15233

412-323-2323

Lehigh County Community College

4525 Education Park Dr.

Schnecksville, PA 28078

610-799-2121

SOUTH CAROLINA

Trident Technical College

P.O. Box 118067

Charleston, SC 29423

803-572-6111

TENNESSEE

Volunteer State Community College

1360 Nashville Pike

Gallatin, TN 37066

615-452-8600

TEXAS

Amarillo College

P.O. Box 447

Amarillo, TX 79178

806-354-6071

Tarrant County Junior College District

1500 Houston St.

Fort Worth, TX 76102

817-336-7851

Houston Community College System

22 Waugh Dr., P.O. Box 7849

Houston, TX 77270

713-869-5021

Transworld Academy, Inc.

6220 W Park Dr.

Houston, TX 77057

713-266-6594

VIRGINIA

Northern Virginia Community College

4001 Wakefield Chapel Rd.

Annandale, VA 22003

703-323-3129

WISCONSIN

Northeast Wisconsin Technical College

2740 W Mason St., P.O. Box 19042

Green Bay, WI 54307

414-498-5400

Milwaukee Area Technical College

700 W State St.

Milwaukee, WI 53233

414-297-6600

RADIOLOGIC TECHNOLOGY

ALABAMA

Jefferson State Community College
2601 Carson Rd.
Birmingham, AL 35215
205-853-1200

Gasden State Community College
P.O. Box 227
Gadsden, AL 35902
205-549-8259

George C. Wallace State Community
College—Hanceville
801 Main St., P.O. Box 2000
Hanceville, AL 35077
205-352-8000

University of Alabama at Birmingham
245 Administration Bldg.
Mobile, AL 36688
205-934-4011

Community College of the Air Force
Maxwell Air Force Base
Montgomery, AL 36112
334-953-6436

ARIZONA

The Bryman School
4343 N 16th St.
Phoenix, AZ 85016
602-274-4300

Gateway Community College
108 N 40th St.
Phoenix, AZ 85034
602-392-5189

ARKANSAS

Sparks Regional Medical Center School of
Radiology
1311 S Eye St.
Fort Smith, AR 72917
501-441-5172

Carti School of Radiation Therapy
Technology
P.O. Box 5210
Little Rock, AR 72215
501-660-7623

Arkansas Valley Technical Institute
Hwy. 23 N, P.O. Box 506
Ozark, AR 72949
501-667-2117

CALIFORNIA

Cabrillo College
6500 Soquel Dr.
Apton, CA 95003
408-479-6461

Orange Coast College
2701 Fairview Rd.
Costa Mesa, CA 92626
714-432-5757

Cypress College
9200 Valley View
Cypress, CA 90630
714-826-2220

Fresno City College
1101 E University Ave.
Fresno, CA 93741
209-442-4600

American School of X-Ray
13723 Harvard Pl.
Gardena, CA 90249
213-770-4001

Loma Linda University
Loma Linda, CA 92350
909-824-4931

Educorp Career College
230 E 3rd St.
Long Beach, CA 90802
310-437-0501

Long Beach City College
4901 E Carson St.
Long Beach, CA 90808
310-420-4176

Foothill College
12345 El Monte Rd.
Los Altos Hills, CA 94022
415-949-7469

Charles R. Drew University of Medicine
and Science
1621 E 120th St.
Los Angeles, CA 90059
213-563-5835

Nova Institute of Health Technology
2400 S Western Ave.
Los Angeles, CA 90018
213-735-2222

Yuba College
2088 N Beale Rd.
Marysville, CA 95901
916-741-6960

Merced College
3600 M St.
Merced, CA 95348
209-384-6132

Modern Technology School of X-Ray
6180 Laurel Canyon Blvd.
North Hollywood, CA 91606
818-763-2563

Butte College
3536 Butte Campus Dr.
Oroville, CA 95965
916-895-2511

Chaffey Community College
5885 Haven Ave.
Rancho Cucamonga, CA 91737
909-941-2359

San Diego Mesa College
7250 Mesa College Dr.
San Diego, CA 92111
619-627-2666

Cancer Foundation Schools of Technology
300 W Pueblo St.
Santa Barbara, CA 93195
805-682-7300

Santa Barbara City College
721 Cliff Dr.
Santa Barbara, CA 93109
805-965-0581

Santa Rosa Junior College
1501 Mendocino Ave.
Santa Rosa, CA 95401
707-527-4346

San Joaquin General Hospital School of
    Radiation Technology
P.O. Box 1020
Stockton, CA 95201
209-468-6233

Mount San Antonio College
1100 N Grand Ave.
Walnut, CA 91789
909-594-5611

Nova Institute of Health Technology
11416 Whittier Blvd.
Whittier, CA 90601
310-695-0771

COLORADO
Community College of Denver
P.O. Box 173363
Denver, CO 80217
303-556-2600

CONNECTICUT
Saint Vincent's Medical Center of
    Nuclear Medicine
2800 Main St.
Bridgeport, CT 06606
203-576-5235

South Central Community College
60 Sargent Dr.
New Haven, CT 06511
203-789-6928

DELAWARE
Delaware Technical and Community College
    Stanton-Wilmington
400 Stanton-Christiana Rd.
Newark, DE 19713
302-454-3900

DISTRICT OF COLUMBIA
George Washington University
2121 I St. NW
Washington, DC 20037
202-994-3725

FLORIDA
Santa Fe Community College
3000 NW 83rd St.
Gainesville, FL 32601
904-395-5702

National School of Technology, Inc.
4355 W 16th Ave.
Hialeah, FL 33012
305-945-2929

Jackson Memorial Medical Center
University of Miami
1611 NW 12th Ave.
Miami, FL 33136
305-585-6811

Florida Hospital College of Health Sciences
800 Lake Estelle Dr.
Orlando, FL 32803
407-895-7747

Palm Beach Community College
3160 PGA Blvd.
Palm Beach Gardens, FL 33410
407-625-2511

Pensacola Junior College
1000 College Blvd.
Pensacola, FL 32504
904-476-5410

Hillsborough Community College
P.O. Box 31127
Tampa, FL 33631
813-253-7004

Saint Petersburg Junior College
P.O. Box 13489
Saint Petersburg, FL 33733
813-546-0021

GEORGIA

Albany Technical Institute
1021 Lowe Rd.
Albany, GA 31708
912-430-3500

Athens Area Technical Institute
899 Hwy. 29 N
Athens, GA 30601
706-542-8050

Emory University School of Medicine
1364 Clifton Rd. NE
Atlanta, GA 30322
404-712-5512

Fulton De Kalb Hospital Authority Grady
   Memorial Hospital
80 Butler St., P.O. Box 26044
Atlanta, GA 30335
404-616-4307

Medical College of Georgia
1120 15th St.
Augusta, GA 30912
706-721-0211

Brunswick College
3700 Altama Ave.
Brunswick, GA 31520
912-264-7235

Medical Center, Inc.—School of Radiologic
   Technology
710 Center St., Hospital Drawer 85
Columbus, GA 31994
404-571-1155

De Kalb Medical Center School of Radiation
   Technology
2701 N Decatur Rd.
Decatur, GA 30033
404-297-5307

HAWAII

Kapiolani Community College
4303 Diamond Head Rd.
Honolulu, HI 96816
808-956-6637

ILLINOIS

Belleville Area College
2500 Carlyle Rd.
Belleville, IL 62221
618-235-2700

Southern Illinois University—Carbondale
Carbondale, IL 62901
618-453-8882

Kaskaskia College
27210 College Rd.
Centralia, IL 62801
618-532-1981

Cook County Hospital School of X-Ray
 Technology
1825 W Harrison St.
Chicago, IL 60612
312-633-8522

College of Du Page
Lambert Rd. and 22nd St.
Glen Ellyn, IL 60137
708-858-2800

Moraine Valley Community College
10900 S 88th Ave.
Paios Hills, IL 60465
708-974-5316

Methodist Medical Center of Illinois—
 Medical Technology
221 NE Glen Oak Ave.
Peoria, IL 61636
309-672-5513

Triton College
2000 5th Ave.
River Grove, IL 60171
708-456-0300

Rockford Memorial Hospital School of
 X-Ray Technology
2400 N Rockton Ave.
Rockford, IL 61103
815-969-5480

Swedish American Hospital School of
 Surgical Technology
1400 Charles St.
Rockford, IL 61104
815-968-4400

INDIANA

Wellborn Cancer Center
401 SE 6th St.
Evansville, IN 47713
812-426-8321

Indiana University—Purdue University
 Indianapolis
355 N Lansing
Indianapolis, IN 46202
317-274-5555

Ball State University
2000 University Ave.
Muncie, IN 48306
765-285-8300

IOWA

Scott Community College
500 Belmont Rd.
Bettendorf, IA 52722
319-359-7531

Jennie Edmundson Memorial Hospital
933 E Pierce St.
Council Bluffs, IA 51503
712-328-6010

Iowa Methodist Medical Center
1200 Pleasant St.
Des Moines, IA 50309
515-241-6171

Iowa Central Community College
1 Triton Cir.
Fort Dodge, IA 50501
515-576-7201

University of Iowa
Iowa City, IA 52242
319-335-3500

KANSAS

Fort Hays State University
600 Park St.
Hays, KS 67601
913-628-4222

Labette Community College
200 S 14th St.
Parsons, KS 67357
620-421-6700

Washburn University of Topeka
1700 College Ave.
Topeka, KS 66621
913-231-1010

KENTUCKY

Kentucky Technical—Bowling Green State
   Vocational Technical School
1845 Loop Dr., P.O. Box 6000
Bowling Green, KY 42101
502-781-0711

Lexington Community College
Cooper Dr.
Lexington, KY 40506
606-257-4831

Morehead State University
150 University Blvd.
Morehead, KY 40351
606-783-2655

LOUISIANA

Delgado Community College
615 City Park Ave.
New Orleans, LA 70119
504-483-4114

MAINE

Southern Maine Technical College
2 Fort Rd.
South Portland, ME 04106
207-767-9520

MARYLAND

Essex Community College
7201 Rossville Rd.
Baltimore, MD 21237
410-780-6363

Prince George's Community College
301 Largo Rd.
Largo, MD 23701
301-322-0819

MASSACHUSETTS

Bunker Hill Community College
250 New Rutherford Ave.
Boston, MA 02129
617-228-2027

Northeastern University
360 Huntington Ave.
Boston, MA 02115
617-373-2525

Massasoit Community College
1 Massasoit Blvd.
Brockton, MA 02402
508-588-9100

Holyoke Community College
303 Homestead Ave.
Holyoke, MA 01040
413-538-7000

Springfield Technical Community College
Armory Square
Springfield, MA 01105
413-781-7822

MICHIGAN

Ferris State University
901 S State Rd.
Big Rapids, MI 49307
616-592-2000

Grand Rapids Community College
143 Bostwick Ave. NE
Grand Rapids, MI 49505
616-456-4965

Lansing Community College
419 N Capitol Ave.
Lansing, MI 48901
517-483-1200

William Beaumont Hospital
3601 W 13 Mile Rd.
Royal Oak, MI 48073
810-551-5000

Carnegie Institute
550 Stephenson Hwy.
Troy, MI 48083
810-589-1078

MINNESOTA

Northwest Technical College—
    East Grand Forks
Hwy. 220 N
East Grand Forks, MN 56721
218-773-3441

Mayo School of Health-Related Sciences
200 1st St. SW
Rochester, MN 55905
507-284-3678

Rochester Community College
851 30th Ave. SE
Rochester, MN 55904
507-285-7210

MISSISSIPPI

University of Mississippi Medical Center
2500 N State St.
Jackson, MS 39216
601-876-3500

MISSOURI

Research Medical Center School of Nuclear
    Medical Technology
2316 E Meyer Blvd.
Kansas City, MO 64132
816-276-3390

Saint Luke's College
4426 Wornall Rd.
Kansas City, MO 64111
816-932-2233

Saint Louis Community College—
Forest Park
5600 Oakland Ave.
Saint Louis, MO 63110
314-644-9280

NEW HAMPSHIRE

New Hampshire Technical Institute
11 Institute Dr.
Concord, NH 03301
603-225-1865

NEW JERSEY

Hudson Area School of Radiologic
Technology
29 E 29th St.
Bayonne, NJ 07002
201-858-5348

Middlesex County College
155 Mill Rd., P.O. Box 3050
Edison, NJ 08818
908-548-6000

University of Medicine and Dentistry of
New Jersey
65 Bergen St.
Newark, NJ 07107
201-982-4821

Bergen Community College
400 Paramus Rd.
Paramus, NJ 07652
201-447-7178

Overlook Hospital School of Nuclear
Medical Technology
99 Beauvoir Ave., P.O. Box 220
Summit, NJ 07902
908-522-2072

NEW YORK

Broome Community College
P.O. Box 1017
Binghamton, NY 13902
607-778-5000

CUNY New York City Technical College
300 Jay St.
Brooklyn, NY 11201
718-260-5560

Trocaire College
110 Red Jackey Pkwy.
Buffalo, NY 14220
716-826-1200

Nassau Community College
1 Education Dr.
Garden City, NY 11530
516-572-7345

Bellevue Hospital Center School of
Radiation Technology
1st Ave. and 27th St.
New York, NY 10016

PENNSYLVANIA

North Hills School of Health Occupations
1500 Northway Mall
Pittsburgh, PA 15237
412-367-8003

Crozer-Chester Medical Center—
  Allied Health Program
1 Medical Center Blvd.
Upland, PA 19013
610-447-2000

Wilkes-Barre General Hospital—School of
  Medical Technology
575 N River St.
Wilkes-Barre, PA 18764
570-829-8111

RHODE ISLAND

Rhode Island Hospital School of Nuclear
  Medicine
593 Eddy St.
Providence, RI 02903
401-444-5724

Community College of Rhode Island
400 East Ave.
Warwick, RI 02886
401-825-1000

SOUTH CAROLINA

Trident Technical College
P.O. Box 118067
Charleston, SC 29423
803-572-6111

Horry-Georgetown Technical College
P.O. Box 1966
Conway, SC 29526
803-347-3186

Greenville Technical College
Station B, P.O. Box 5616
Greenville, SC 29606
803-250-8000

TENNESSEE

Chattanooga State Technical Community
  College
4501 Amnicola Hwy.
Chattanooga, TN 37406
423-697-4400

Roane State Community College
276 Patton Ln.
Harriman, TN 37748
615-882-4501

East Tennessee State University
P.O. Box 70716
Johnson City, TN 37614
423-929-4112

Shelby State Community College
P.O. Box 40568
Memphis, TN 38174
901-544-5000

TEXAS

Amarillo College
P.O. Box 447
Amarillo, TX 79178
806-354-6071

Austin Community College
5930 Middle Fiskville Rd.
Austin, TX 78782
512-223-7504

Lamar University—Beaumont
4400 MLK, P.O. Box 10001
Beaumont, TX 77710
409-880-8845

El Centro College
Main and Lamar
Dallas, TX 75202
214-746-2278

El Paso Community College
P.O. Box 20500
El Paso, TX 79998
915-594-2000

Moncrief Radiation Center School of
    Radiation Therapy
1450 8th Ave.
Fort Worth, TX 76104
817-923-7393

Galveston College
4015 Ave. Q
Galveston, TX 77550
409-772-9467

Houston Community College System
22 Waugh Dr., P.O. Box 7849
Houston, TX 77270
713-869-5021

Ultrasound Diagnostic School
580 Decker Drive
Irving, TX 75062
214-791-1120

San Jacinto College—Central Campus
8060 Spencer Hwy.
Pasadena, TX 77505
713-476-1871

Saint Philip's College
1801 Martin Luther King Dr.
San Antonio, TX 78203
512-531-3591

McLennan Community College
1400 College Dr.
Waco, TX 76708
817-750-3542

Midwestern State University
3410 Taft Blvd.
Wichita Falls, TX 76308
817-689-4608

UTAH
Utah Valley Hospital School of Radiologic
    Technology
1034 N 5th West St.
Provo, UT 84603
801-373-7850

VIRGINIA
Tidewater Community College
Rte. 135
Portsmouth, VA 23703
804-484-2121

WASHINGTON
Bellevue Community College
3000 Landerholm Cir. SE
Bellevue, WA 98007
206-641-0111

Tacoma Community College
5900 S 12th St.
Tacoma, WA 98465
206-756-5000

Yakima Valley Community College
P.O. Box 1647
Yakima, WA 98907
509-575-2373

WEST VIRGINIA

West Virginia University Hospital School of
   Radiation Technology
Medical Center Dr., P.O. Box 8062
Morgantown, WV 26506
304-598-4252

WISCONSIN

Milwaukee Area Technical College
700 W State St.
Milwaukee, WI 53233
414-297-6600

Saint Joseph's Hospital School of Medical
   Technology
611 Saint Joseph's Ave.
Marshfield, WI 54449
715-387-7202

Saint Luke's Medical Center School of
   Diagnostic Medical Sonography
2900 W Oklahoma Ave.
Milwaukee, WI 53215
414-649-6762

Mercy Medical Center School of Radiologic
   Technology
631 Hazel St.
Oshkosh, WI 54902
414-236-2253

SURGICAL TECHNOLOGY

ALABAMA

Community College of the Air Force
Maxwell Air Force Base
Montgomery, AL 36112
334-953-6436

ARIZONA

The Bryman School
4343 N 16th St.
Phoenix, AZ 85016
602-274-4300

CALIFORNIA

California Paramedic and Technical College
3745 Long Beach Blvd.
Long Beach, CA 90807
310-595-6630

Institute of Business and Medical Technology
75-110 St. Charles Place
Palm Desert, CA 92260
818-597-8490

Newbridge College
700 El Camino Real
Tustin, CA 92680
714-573-8787

COLORADO

Concorde Career Institute

770 Grant St.

Denver, CO 80203

303-861-1151

FLORIDA

Sheridan Vocational Center

5400 W Sheridan St.

Hollywood, FL 33021

954-985-3220

GEORGIA

Athens Area Technical Institute

800 Hwy. 29 N

Athens, GA 30601

706-542-8050

ILLINOIS

Swedish American Hospital School of
    Surgical Technology

1400 Charles St.

Rockford, IL 61104

815-968-4400

KENTUCKY

Kentucky Department for Adult & Technical
    Education—Central Kentucky SVTS

104 Vo-Tech Rd.

Lexington, KY 40510

606-255-8501

Kentucky Technical—Jefferson State
    Vocational Technical School

727 W Chestnut St.

Louisville, KY 40203

502-595-4221

LOUISIANA

Delgado Community College

615 City Park Ave.

New Orleans, LA 70119

504-483-4114

MASSACHUSETTS

New England Baptist Hospital School
    of Nursing

220 Fisher Ave.

Boston, MA 02120

617-739-5260

Quincy College

34 Coddington St.

Quincy, MA 02169

617-984-1600

MICHIGAN

Lansing Community College

419 N Capitol Ave.

Lansing, MI 48901

517-483-9850

MINNESOTA

Northwest Technical College—East Grand
    Forks

Hwy. 220 N

East Grand Forks, MN 56721

218-773-3441

Minnesota Riverland Technical College—
    Rochester Campus

1926 College View Rd. SE

Rochester, MN 55904

507-285-8631

Saint Cloud Technical College
1540 Northway Dr.
Saint Cloud MN 56303
612-654-5000

MISSISSIPPI

Itawamba Community College
602 W Hill St.
Fulton, MS 38843
601-862-3101

PENNSYLVANIA

Mount Aloysius College
1 College Dr.
Cresson, PA 16630-1999
814-886-4131

Delaware County Community College
901 S Media Line Rd.
Media, PA 19063
610-359-5000

Saint Francis Medical Center School
   of Nursing
400 45th St.
Pittsburgh, PA 15201
412-622-4494

Wilkes-Barre General Hospital—School of
   Medical Technology
North River and Auburn
Wilkes-Barre, PA 18764
717-820-2737

SOUTH CAROLINA

Midlands Technical College
P.O. Box 2408
Columbia, SC 29202
803-738-8324

York Technical College
452 S Anderson Rd.
Rock Hill, SC 29730
803-327-8000

TENNESSEE

Knoxville State Area Vocational-Technical
   School
1100 Liberty St.
Knoxville, TN 37919
423-546-5568

Memphis Area Vocational Technical School
550 Alabama Ave.
Memphis, TN 38105
901-543-6100

Aquinas Junior College
4210 Harding Rd.
Nashville, TN 37205
615-297-7545

TEXAS

Texas State Technical College—Harlingen
   Campus
1902 N Loop
Harlingen, TX 78550
956-364-4000

Houston Community College System
22 Waugh Dr., P.O. Box 7849
Houston, TX 77270
713-869-5021

South Plains College
1401 College Ave.
Levelland, TX 79336
806-894-9611

San Antonio College of Medical and Dental
  Assistants
5280 Medical Dr.
San Antonio, TX 78229
210-692-0241

Temple Junior College
2600 S 1st St.
Temple, TX 76504
817-773-9961

VIRGINIA

NNPS RRMC School of Surgical Technology
12420 Warwick Blvd.
Newport News, VA 23606
757-594-2722

WASHINGTON

Seattle Central Community College
1701 Broadway
Seattle, WA 98122
206-587-3800

WISCONSIN

Northeast Wisconsin Technical Center
2740 W Mason St., P.O. Box 19042
Green Bay, WI 54307
414-498-5400

CHAPTER four

FINANCIAL AID FOR THE TRAINING YOU NEED

MANY POTENTIAL students think they cannot afford college because of the high costs. It may cost $25,000 or more a year to go to a major university. Before you attend a training school or college, you must figure out whether you can afford classes, books, and any extracurricular activities you want to take. You should also explore the financial aid opportunities that are available to help you pay for the training program you want.

THIS CHAPTER explains how to receive financial aid from the school you wish to attend. You will find information on how to gather your financial records, determine your eligibility for financial aid, distinguish between different types of financial aid, and file your forms once you have completed them. Sample financial aid forms and interviews from financial aid advisors and students who have received aid will help guide you through the process.

TYPES OF FINANCIAL AID

Many types of financial aid are available to help with school expenses. Most financial aid is determined by need. There are loans, which you have to pay back after your schooling is through, and there are grants and scholarships, which you do not have to pay back. Grants and any outside scholarships will be factored in to your application profile to determine whether you require any interest-bearing loans. For more detailed information about each type of assistance, see your financial aid counselor and refer to the financial aid booklet you receive with your application.

Scholarships

Amazingly enough, you can attend a small college or even a university without paying a dime if you know what to do and if you can establish adequate financial need. One nursing student from Dallas, Texas, explains how she did it:

> *I researched carefully what kind of aid I might be eligible to receive. I have a small child, so I knew my expenses would be tight. I applied for and received the Pell Grant and the Hope Scholarship. Between the two types of aid, I have money left over for books and some daycare expenses. I work part time for money to live on day to day, but I am getting an education basically tuition-free.*

There are thousands and thousands of scholarship dollars available out there for aspiring students—many institutions offer scholarships that most students do not know about. If you do your research, you will most likely be able to apply for and possibly earn a good chunk of money (which you are not required to pay back after your schooling is through!). Every state has specific scholarships available for residents, and private scholarships from organizations are also awarded on a regular basis. For more information on scholarships, contact your financial aid counselor, who should have a comprehensive list to share with you during your application process. See the Appendix for addresses of scholarships listed below.

Examples of state scholarships include but are not limited to the following.

▶ The Hope Scholarship is a Georgia lottery–funded scholarship for Georgia-resident students who maintain at least a 3.0 GPA.

- ▶ The New Hampshire Charitable Foundation offers scholarships to New Hampshire residents.
- ▶ The Illinois Hospital Association Scholarship is offered to Illinois residents with a 3.5 GPA or higher.
- ▶ The Allied Healthcare Scholarship Program awards scholarships to California students with a 2.0 GPA or higher who commit to a one-year service obligation or 100 to 150 hours of volunteer service practicing direct patient care in a medically underserved area (MUA) of California.
- ▶ The Procter & Gamble American College of Prosthodontists Research Fellowship is available to dental students, residents, fellows, and graduate students enrolled in U.S. schools of dentistry in dental-related fields. Applicants must submit a research proposal to be eligible for this award.
- ▶ The American Medical Technologists Student Scholarship is available to high school seniors and current college students enrolled in a field of study that will lead to a career in medical technology or a related field.

Military scholarships are also available if you are applying to the Army, Navy, Air Force, or Marines; these scholarships include the G.I. Bill and other money for college or to pay off previous loans.

Private scholarships, such as the following, are also available.

- ▶ The Maxine Williams Scholarships are awarded by the American Association of Medical Assistants Endowment.
- ▶ The American Medical Technologist Scholarship awards $250 to high school students or graduates in good standing.
- ▶ The American Association of Homes for the Aging offers Nurse Education Scholarships.
- ▶ The Dental Assisting Scholarship Program, part of the ADA Endowment Fund and Assistance, offers scholarships.
- ▶ The Mary Catherine Smalley Memorial Scholarship offers scholarships to nursing students with a 3.0 GPA or higher at Worcester State College.

▶ The Pfizer Consumer Healthcare scholarships is offered to dental hygiene students with a 3.0 GPA or higher enrolled in an accredited program in the United States.

▶ The Pinnacle Healthcare Scholarship is offered to students at Arizona Western College who have a 2.0 GPA or higher.

▶ The St. David's Neal Kocurek Scholarship is offered to students in Hays, Travis, and Williamson, Texas.

A financial aid counselor from William Paterson College in New Jersey says:

I get notice of many scholarships for health careers. I publish them in the school paper and on the TV and radio stations on campus. I also refer students to the nursing department, which posts scholarships sent directly there. Schools also offer minority scholarships, trustee scholarships, and presidential scholarships. The state of New Jersey offers the Garden State Scholarship for Garden State distinguished scholars. The college will match you to the available scholarships. Deadline dates are important. The most important thing you can do for yourself is apply early.

Federal Pell Grants

Unlike a loan, a Federal Pell Grant does not have to be repaid. Pell Grants are need-based grants awarded to undergraduate students who have not yet earned a bachelor's or professional degree and students enrolled in certain post-baccalaureate programs that lead to teacher certification or licensure. For many students, Pell Grants provide a foundation of financial aid to which other aid may be added.

Awards for the award year will depend on program funding. The maximum award for the 2008–2009 award year was $4,731. You can receive only one Pell Grant in an award year. The amount you receive will depend not only on your expected family contribution (EFC) but also on your cost of attendance, whether you are a full-time or part-time student, and whether you attend school for a full academic year or less. You cannot receive Pell Grant funds for more than one school at a time.

Federal Supplemental Educational Opportunity Grants (FSEOG)

An FSEOG is for undergraduates with exceptional financial need—that is, students with the lowest EFCs—and gives priority to students who receive Federal Pell Grants. An FSEOG does not have to be paid back.

You can receive between $100 and $4,000 a year, depending on when you apply, your level of need, and the funding level of the school you are attending. There is no guarantee that every eligible student will be able to receive an FSEOG. Students at each school are paid based on the availability of funds at that school; not all schools participate in the program.

Federal Work-Study Program

The Federal Work-Study Program provides jobs for undergraduate and graduate students with financial need and allows them to earn money to help pay education expenses. The program encourages community service work and provides hands-on experience related to your course of study.

Your work-study salary will be at least the current federal minimum wage or higher, depending on the type of work you do and the skills required. Your total award depends on when you apply, your level of need, and the funding level of your school. The average new award for the 2008–2009 award year was $1,478. Not all schools have work-study in every area of study.

Federal Perkins Loans

A Federal Perkins Loan has the lowest interest rate (5%) of any loan available for both undergraduate and graduate students with exceptional financial need. Your school is your lender, and the loan is made with government funds. You must repay this loan to your school within the 10-year repayment period.

Depending on when you apply, your level of need, and the funding level of the school, you can borrow up to $5,500 for each year of undergraduate study and up to $8,000 for each year of graduate study. The cumulative total you can borrow as an undergraduate is $27,500. The cumulative total you can borrow for undergraduate and graduate study combined is $60,000.

After graduating, if you gain employment in certain public, military, or teaching service positions, you may be eligible to have all or part of your loans canceled. Your financial aid administrator can work with you to determine your eligibility.

Parental Loans for Undergraduate Students (PLUS) Loans

PLUS loans enable parents with good credit histories to borrow money to pay education expenses of a child who is a dependent undergraduate student enrolled at least half time in an eligible program at an eligible school. PLUS loans are available through both the Direct Loan and FFEL programs (explained in the next section). Your parents must submit the completed forms to your school.

To be eligible, your parents will be required to pass a credit check. If they do not pass the credit check, they may still be able to receive a loan if they can prove extenuating circumstances or if someone who is able to pass the credit check agrees to cosign the loan. Your parents must also meet citizenship requirements.

The yearly limit on a PLUS Loan is equal to your cost of attendance minus any other financial aid you receive. For instance, if your cost of attendance is $10,000 and you receive $6,000 in other financial aid, your parents can borrow up to, but no more than, $4,000.

Direct and Federal Family Education Loan (FFEL) Stafford Loans

Direct and FFEL Stafford Loans are a major form of financial aid. Direct Stafford Loans are available through the William D. Ford Federal Direct

Loan Program, and FFEL Stafford Loans are available through the FFEL Program. The major differences between the two are the source of the loan funds, some aspects of the application process, and the available repayment plans.

Direct and FFEL Stafford Loans are either subsidized or unsubsidized. A subsidized loan is awarded on the basis of financial need. You will not be charged any interest before you begin repayment or during authorized periods of deferment. The federal government subsidizes the interest during these periods.

An unsubsidized loan is not awarded on the basis of need. You will be charged interest from the time the loan is disbursed until it is paid in full. If you allow the interest to accumulate, it will be capitalized—that is, the interest will be added to the principal amount of your loan, and additional interest will be based on the higher amount. This will increase the amount you have to repay.

If you are a dependent undergraduate student, you can borrow up to the following amounts:

▶ $5,500 a year if you are a first-year student enrolled in a program that is at least a full academic year (no more than $3,500 of this amount may be in subsidized loans)

▶ $6,500 a year if you have completed your first year of study and the remainder of your program is at least a full academic year (no more than $4,500 of this amount may be in subsidized loans)

▶ $7,500 a year if you have completed two years of study and the remainder of your program is at least a full academic year (no more than $5,500 of this amount may be in subsidized loans)

If you are an independent undergraduate student or a dependent student whose parents are unable to get a PLUS Loan, you may borrow up to the following amounts:

▶ $9,500 a year if you are a first-year student enrolled in a program that is at least a full academic year (no more than $3,500 of this amount may be in subsidized loans)

▶ $10,500 a year if you have completed your first year of study and the remainder of your program is at least a full academic year (no more than $4,500 of this amount may be in subsidized loans)

▶ $12,500 a year if you have completed two years of study and the remainder of your program is at least a full academic year (no more than $5,500 of this amount may be in subsidized loans)

▶ $20,500 a year if you are a graduate or professional degree student (no more than $8,500 of this amount may be in subsidized loans)

Loan Repayment

If you receive any interest-bearing student loans, after graduation you will attend exit counseling, during which the lenders will tell you your total debt and work out a payment schedule with you. Many loans include a grace period, so you need not start paying them off for at least six to nine months after you graduate. For example, you do not have to begin repaying the Perkins Loan until nine months after you graduate. This grace period gives you time to find a job and start earning money. During this time, you may have to pay the interest on your loan.

Repayment schedules differ according to your salary. You may begin repaying the highest amount available or opt for a graduated repayment schedule. A graduated repayment schedule allows you to start with small payments that will increase as your salary level increases. If for some reason you remain unemployed when your payments become due, you may receive an unemployment deferment for a certain length of time. For many of these loans, you will have a maximum repayment period of 10 years (excluding periods of deferment and forbearance).

Consolidating Loans for Repayment

A consolidation loan is designed to help student and parent borrowers simplify loan repayment by allowing the borrower to consolidate several types of federal student loans with various repayment schedules into one loan.

The interest rate on the consolidation loan may be lower than what you are currently paying on one or more of your loans. Financial administrators recommend that you do not consolidate a Perkins Loan with any other loans since the interest on a Perkins Loan is already the lowest available.

GETTING STARTED

Every school has a financial aid department. This is where you can obtain a financial aid application called the Free Application for Federal Student Aid (FAFSA). The FAFSA is the form used by the U.S. Department of Education to determine your EFC by conducting a *need analysis* based on financial information, such as income, assets, and other household information, which you (and your parents if you are a dependent student) will be asked to provide. The form is submitted to, and processed by, a federal processor contracted by the U.S. Department of Education, and the results are electronically transmitted to the financial aid offices of the schools that you list on your application.

The FAFSA application is used by nearly all colleges and universities to determine eligibility for federal, state, and college-sponsored financial aid, including grants, educational loans, and work-study programs. You should make it a high priority to complete this application; it determines your eligibility status for all grants and loans provided by federal or state governments and certain college or institution aid.

Nearly every student is eligible for some form of financial aid, including low-interest Federal Stafford and/or PLUS loans, regardless of income or circumstances, provided that you

- are a U.S. citizen, a U.S. national, or an eligible noncitizen
- have a valid social security number
- have a high school diploma or GED
- are registered with the U.S. Selective Service (if you are a male aged 18 to 25)
- complete a FAFSA promising to use any federal aid for educational purposes
- do not owe refunds on any federal student grants

▶ are not in default on any student loans

▶ have not been found guilty of the sale or possession of illegal drugs during a period in which you received federal aid

To receive an application in the mail, contact the U.S. Department of Education at 800-433-3242 or on the web at www.ed.gov. You can also file your FAFSA application online and review eligibility requirements at www.fafsa.com.

The U.S. Department of Education website offers a host of free resources to help you explore your financial aid options.

▶ applications and guidelines for approximately 200 different grant programs

▶ *Guide to Education Programs*, an annual online publication that provides information on financial assistance offered to state and local education agencies, institutions of higher education, other postsecondary institutions, public and private nonprofit organizations, and individuals.

▶ the *FAFSA4caster*, which provides you with an early estimate of how much aid you might be eligible for. It also explains the basics of the federal student aid programs and the application process.

▶ relevant publications such as *Student Guide and Funding Your Education*

More on Scholarships

There are many scholarships available to students in every area of the country. By spending time and energy on a diligent scholarship search, you may be able to attain a higher level of education than you originally thought you could afford. The potential benefits to your professional and personal growth are almost limitless.

One good place to start your scholarship search is at www.studentaid .ed.gov. You can download free publications, review a scholarship checklist, and utilize a free scholarship search service to search by occupation or keyword for federal and private scholarships.

MyFSA is a personal online portfolio you can set up at www.student aid.ed.gov to help you manage your scholarship search and get the most benefit from your time. Once you begin a financial aid application, MyFSA will track where you stopped entering your information and will link you to all applications in progress. It will also provide the date and confirmation number of your submitted applications. You can select colleges you are interested in attending and add them to your MyFSA. Any colleges you add to MyFSA will be stored in and accessed through this area. These colleges will automatically be used in worksheets and tables calling for colleges. You may add or delete colleges from this list at any time.

Once you have completed the Self-Assessment and Career Finder, any careers or majors that have met your specifications can be stored and accessed here. The information you enter about yourself will be stored in your profile. Make sure to keep your information as accurate and up-to-date as possible.

Using the Financial Aid Wizard, you can store and access any scholarships, loans, and cost of attendance information. You can even calculate an EFC. (This section of MyFSA uses the same schools shown in the Colleges section earlier in this chapter to calculate approximate costs. At your option, profile information can be used to prepopulate certain fields on the FAFSA, FAFSA4caster, and electronic college admission applications.

It is easy to find online resources to help you search for scholarships. Here are just a few:

http://apps.collegeboard.com
www.findtuition.com
www.naacp.org
www.getscholarshipmoney.com

Other sources of scholarship awards that are worth pursuing include local hospitals, colleges, or institutions; large businesses; your employer; community and religious organizations; special interest groups; and minority advocacy organizations.

Determining Your Eligibility

To receive financial aid from an accredited college or institution's student aid program, you must:

▶ show proof of financial need, except for some loan programs (Since you agree to pay loans back with interest, most loan programs do not require proof of financial need. Some smaller schools, with smaller loaning pools, may require proof of need.)

▶ have a high school diploma or a GED certificate, pass a test approved by the U.S. Department of Education, or meet other standards your state establishes that are approved by the U.S. Department of Education

▶ be enrolled or accepted for enrollment as a regular student working toward a degree or certificate in an eligible program

▶ be a U.S. citizen or an eligible noncitizen

▶ have a valid social security number

▶ make satisfactory academic progress during the time you are receiving financial aid

▶ sign a statement of educational purpose and a certification statement on overpayment and default

▶ register with selective services, if required

When to Apply

Much of the federal financial aid is available on a first-come, first-served basis. You should file your application early to increase your chances of receiving the maximum financial aid you qualify for.

You can apply for financial aid after January 1 of the year in which you want to enroll. For example, if you want to begin school in the fall of 2012, you should apply for financial aid as soon as possible after January 1, 2012. **Note:** If you apply online at www.fafsa.com, you may submit your application on the website before January 1, and FAFSA will file it for you automatically on January 1, which would put you ahead of other people who delay filing their application.

It is easier to complete the application when you already have your completed tax return, so if you are not someone's dependent and are in charge of your own finances, consider filing your taxes as early as possible as well. If you apply by mail, send your completed application in the envelope that came with it. The envelope is already addressed, and using it will ensure that your application reaches the correct address.

Do not forget that **you must reapply for financial aid every year**. However, after your first year, you will receive a Student Aid Report (SAR) from the federal government before the application deadline. If it needs no corrections, you can just sign it and send it in. On your financial aid application you can request to receive your SAR either electronically or through the postal mail.

Many students lose out on thousands of dollars in grants and loans because they file too late. A financial aid counselor from William Paterson College in New Jersey suggests:

> *When you fill out the Free Application for Federal Student Aid (FAFSA), you are applying for all aid available, both federal and state, work-study, student loans, etc. The important thing is complying with the deadline date. Those students who do are considered for the Pell Grant, the SEOG (Supplemental Educational Opportunity Grant), and the Perkins Loan, which is the best loan as far as interest goes. Lots of students miss the deadline, and it can mean losing thousands of dollars that they would have qualified to receive. Unfortunately, students, usually the ones who need the money most, often ignore the deadlines.*

Getting Your Forms Filed

Filing your forms is as simple as remembering the following three things:

▶ Pay attention to the deadlines. Some deadlines are as early as the second week in January. Visit www.fafsa.com for a current database of state deadlines.

▶ Pay attention to the details. Different colleges word their deadline instructions differently, so check deadline details carefully. For example, does the financial aid application deadline refer to the date by which you must submit your FAFSA application or is it the date by which your completed financial aid application must be received in the college financial aid office from the federal processor? You need to know.

▶ Fill out the forms as completely as possible. Make an appointment with a financial aid counselor or consult a FAFSA Student Aid Advisor if you need help.

FAFSA offers two electronic filing options:

1. Call 866-514-5948 to speak with a Student Aid Advisor who will guide you through the application (expect to spend 15 to 20 minutes on the phone), check your application for accuracy, and file it for you electronically.

2. Log onto www.fafsa.com to file your application yourself on a secure website. A Student Aid Advisor will then review your application and submit it to the federal processor.

Many financial aid counselors complain that students do not read the forms completely and do not file early enough. Your success in your career depends on how serious you are about working toward your goal, and this is the first of many steps you will take toward working in the healthcare world. Treat it as seriously as you will soon treat your school work. Securing financial aid is an important step toward your goal, so put some time and your best effort into this process. It can make the difference between being able to attend school and not being able to afford an education.

If you apply electronically through a school's website or the FAFSA website, your application will be processed in about a week. If you apply by mail, your application will be processed in approximately four weeks. Then you will receive your SAR. The SAR will report the information from your application, and if there are no questions or problems with your application, your SAR will report your EFC, the number used in determining your eligibility for federal student aid. Each school you list on the application also will get your financial application information if the school is able to receive the information electronically. Check with the schools to which you are applying to make sure they are equipped to receive electronic files. If not, you will have to send them the information yourself via regular mail.

Financial Need

Aid from most of the programs discussed in this chapter is awarded on the basis of financial need (except unsubsidized Stafford and all PLUS and consolidation loans). When you apply for federal student aid, the information you report is used in a formula established by the U.S. Congress. The formula determines your EFC, the amount you and your family are expected to contribute toward your education. If your EFC is below a certain amount, you'll be eligible for a Federal Pell Grant, assuming you meet all other eligibility requirements.

There is no maximum EFC that defines eligibility for the other financial aid options. Instead, your EFC is used in an equation to determine your financial needs.

$$\text{Cost of attendance} - \text{EFC} = \text{Financial Need}$$

A financial aid administrator calculates your cost of attendance and subtracts the amount you and your family are expected to contribute toward that cost. If anything is left over, you are considered to have financial need.

Gathering Financial Records

Your financial need for grants or loans depends on your financial standing. When you apply for aid, your answers to certain questions will determine whether you are considered dependent on your parents, in which case you must report their income and assets as well as your own, or independent, in which case you must report only your own income and assets (and those of your spouse if you are married).

You are considered to be an independent student if at least one of the following applies to you:

▶ you are at least 24 years old
▶ you are married
▶ you have legal dependents other than a spouse
▶ you are an orphan or ward of the court (or were a ward of the court until age 18)
▶ you are a member or a veteran of the U.S. Armed Forces
▶ you are a graduate or a professional degree student

If you live with your parents and if they claimed you as a dependent on their last tax return, then your need will be based on your parents' income. Students are classified as dependent or independent because federal student aid programs are based on the idea that students (and their parents or spouse, if applicable) have the primary responsibility for paying for their postsecondary education.

You will need to gather your tax records for the year prior to the year for which you are applying. For example, if you apply for the fall of 2012, you will use your tax records from 2011.

HELPFUL TELEPHONE NUMBERS AND WEBSITES

If you need immediate answers to questions about federal student aid or application forms, call the hotline number 800-433-3243 at the Federal Student Aid Information Center between 9 A.M. and 8 P.M. (Eastern time), Monday through Friday. If you are hearing impaired, call 800-730-8913, a toll-free TDD (telecommunication device for the deaf) number at the Information Center.

The Student Guide is also available online at the Department of Education's web address: www.ed.gov/prog_info/SFAStudentGuide.

Help in completing the FAFSA is available online too, at www.ed.gov/prog_info/SFA\FAFSA.

A list of Title IV school codes that you may need to complete the FAFSA is available at www.ed.gov/offices/OPE/t4_codes.html.

The following phone numbers and websites may be of help as you fill out your forms:

Selective Service: 888-655-1825; TTY (text telephone): 847-688-2567; www.ss.gov

U.S. Citizenship and Immigration Services: 800-375-5283; TTY: 800-767-1833; www.uscis.gov

Internal Revenue Service: 800-829-1040; TDD: 800-829-4059; www.irs.gov

Social Security Administration: 800-772-1213; TTY: 800-325-0778; www.ssa.gov

National Merit Scholarship Corporation: 847-866-5100; www.nationalmerit.org

Sallie Mae (Student Loan Marketing Association): 888-272-5543; TDD: 888-833-7562; www.salliemae.com

THE INSIDE TRACK

Who: James Baker

What: Radiologic technology student

Where: Carti School of Radiation Therapy Technology,
              Little Rock, Arkansas

INSIDER'S ADVICE

I was 24 when I went back to school, so I wasn't dependent on my parents, but I didn't have much money of my own either. I applied for financial aid as soon as I found out which school I was applying to. I knew I probably wouldn't get a grant because I worked part time and I didn't have any dependents. I thought the best chance I'd have was to get a low-interest loan. I received an unsubsidized Stafford loan.

Since I was working part time, I didn't need the whole amount they offered. I asked if I could take only what I needed, so I wouldn't owe so much money and interest after school. I figured out my school expenses and my living expenses, and my financial aid advisor and I came up with a reasonable borrowing amount. My advice is to do the same. Do not borrow more than you need and end up putting yourself into major debt. An unsubsidized loan gathers interest as long as you have it. I began paying the interest as I made a little extra money from work. This means my debt will be lower when I finish school.

INSIDER'S FUTURE

I want to get a good job as a radiologic technologist at a reputable hospital when I finish my certificate training. I'm not sure what I will do after that. My future is still pretty open to suggestion. I became interested in radiology after I had an accident that caused head trauma. I wanted to be able to understand the x-ray and be able to explain what I was looking at. Once I begin working and finally pay off my loan, I may go back to school, or who knows where I may end up.

CHAPTER five

HOW TO LAND YOUR FIRST JOB

THIS CHAPTER explains how to land your first job after your training program. First you will learn how to conduct your job search, from researching the field to using online resources, classified ads, hotlines, job fairs, and industry publications. Then you will find advice on how to write your resume and cover letter and how to ace your interview. To help you through interviews, which for some people can be the most stressful aspect of the job search, there are tips on advance preparation, answering any tough questions that might be thrown your way, and demonstrating your knowledge in the most effective way possible. Next is information on networking, including ways to make and maintain networking contacts throughout your career. You will also find testimonials from career counselors, employment recruiters, and workers who have advice on landing a job.

YOU CAN begin seeking employment while still in school, if you are not too far from graduation and any certification you need. There are many ways to conduct your job search, from posting your resume online to sending out a slew of resumes. Read on for the latest information on how to land a great job in the healthcare field.

CONDUCTING YOUR JOB SEARCH

The more positions you apply for, the better your chances of landing a job. Try not to apply to only one or two jobs; instead, put yourself out there through several avenues and see what opportunities arise. Keep in mind that major cities usually offer more employment opportunities than smaller towns or cities; your location has a lot to do with the number and variety of jobs that will be available. Also, try not to get discouraged if you do not find something right away. Most job seekers apply for a number of openings before they find employment, especially when the job market is suffering and the economy in general is slow.

Online Resources

The Internet has become a great place to scout for healthcare jobs. Multiple online career centers offer classified ads and jobs within specific careers that are updated daily for qualified applicants. For example, www.careermosaic.com and www.jobweb.org offer numerous job listings in the healthcare field, from nurses to medical assistants.

Health magazine and newsgroup web pages, such as www.healthgate.com and www.medsearch.com, also advertise jobs. Some hospitals and companies also have web pages that list job openings, such as www.medctr.ucla.edu/ (UCLA Medical Center) and www.reidhosp.com (Reid Hospital and Health Care Services in Richmond, Indiana). Start your search with keywords such as *hospitals*, *health*, and *medical centers*, or search for the name of a particular hospital or medical center to see whether it has a website listed. See the list of web addresses below for more job-related websites.

Healthcare Job Search Sites
www.allhealthjobs.com
www.health-care.careerbuilder.com
www.healthcarejobs.org
www.healthjobsstarthere.com
www.healthjobsusa.com
www.medhunters.com
www.nursingjobs.org

General Job Search Sites

www.careermosaic.com

www.careersite.com

www.jobbankusa.com

www.jobsource.com

www.jobweb.com

www.monster.com

Help Wanted Ads

One way to search for a job is by reading the classified advertisements in your local newspapers, trade journals, and professional magazines. Trade journals and professional magazines are not only a good place to find advertisements, but also a useful source of information on current medical trends, institution expansions, large group hirings, and job fairs.

When you find openings that interest you, follow up on each ad by the method requested. You may be asked to phone or send a resume. Always take care to follow directions—if an ad specifies that they prefers emails and not phone calls, pay attention! Record the date of your follow-up, and if you do not hear from the employer within two or three weeks, place another call or send a polite note to the contact on the ad asking whether the job is still open.

An occupational assistant from San Francisco, California, explains how he got his job through a classified ad:

> *I found my current job by answering a want ad in the San Francisco Observer. It was not the first job for which I tried to get an interview through the newspaper. The ad said to call, so I did, and I was given an interview date and time. I dressed up in a jacket and tie for the interview, and I must have impressed them. They interviewed five others for the job, but two weeks later I was hired. I had a 90-day probationary period, so if things didn't work out, either they or I could terminate the employment within that time.*

Career Services

Most vocational schools, high schools, and colleges have a **placement or career service center**. If you are a student or a recent graduate, you should check these resources for job leads first. Many employers look to recruit employees from technical or trade schools and colleges. They may hold job fairs and conduct on-campus interviews with students. The career or guidance counselor at your school should have up-to-date job listings, and might even have connections in the healthcare field from having placed former students (who perhaps went on to be successful employees!) in previous years.

Local and state employment services are another source of information for job openings. There are thousands of such offices in the nation, and many employers automatically list their job openings at the local office. You can search for employment offices by state at www.job-hunt.org. Whether you are seeking a job in private industry or with the state, these offices, which are affiliated with the federal employment service, are worth contacting.

Employment services, or agencies, serve as intermediaries between workers and employers, with the stated goal of matching the companies' needs with the workers' skills and interests. Employment agencies may be privately owned or sponsored by state or federal labor departments. Employment agencies, especially those sponsored by state governments, have enough personnel to process thousands of applications, unlike the companies' own human resource departments. Unemployed workers are strongly encouraged to visit employment agencies and fill out numerous applications.

Employment agencies also maintain a database of skilled, semiskilled, and unskilled workers available for hire. Whenever a potential employer posts a specific job opening with the agency, all of the registered applicants with matching skills may receive a phone call or a postal card notifying them of this opening. Staff members of employment agencies may conduct a mini-interview or give interested applicants more details about the position. Sometimes the only message will be an address and contact information, and it is up to the applicant to make arrangements for an interview directly with the potential employer.

Private employment agencies perform many of the same services, but they are less likely to be overworked and understaffed. Applicants fill out detailed information sheets, covering all of their marketable skills and employment experiences. In addition, applicants may also receive training in resume writing, interviewing skills, and presentation. Some aptitude testing may also be available to determine the applicant's strongest skills.

Private employment agencies will help you get a job if they think they can place you. Most employment agencies get paid by a company only if they place you in a job at that company, so you need to show the agency that you are a good prospect. Agency staff will help you prepare a resume if you need one, and they will contact employers they think might be interested in you. Some may require a small registration fee whether or not you get a job through them. Private employment agencies may have established relationships with local employers, making it easier for applicants to get past the first round of screenings. Private employment agencies may also offer temporary job services, allowing workers to earn survival money until something more lucrative or satisfying becomes available. Temporary job assignments may involve menial labor in a factory setting or entry-level clerical work such as data entry or filing. As useful as these services may be, private employment agencies can charge you a fee for the privilege of having your name listed in their database. It pays to ask questions before entering into a contract with private employment agencies. Never fall for promises of high-paying jobs with little or no experience required.

Employment agencies should be seen as supplemental sources for your job search, not necessarily as your only option. Finding work through employment agencies is often a numbers game—hundreds of other applicants may have received the same job leads, so be prepared for screenings and interviews.

You can access **career services online** at sites like those listed earlier under the heading Online Resources. Many of those sites offer free online career screening and placement services. Once you register, you may post your resume or employment profile to a secure website. When companies that subscribe to the service have a job to fill, they can call up a certain combination of qualifications on their computer system and quickly receive information on appropriate candidate(s). Most of these sites give you the option of marking your resume and profile either public or private. If you mark it public, your information will be visible to all visitors to the site. This increases your exposure to potential employers and may generate more interest. If you mark your information private, your profile will be viewable only to site subscribers. This affords you an extra level of privacy, but also reduces the pool of potential employers who can find you.

Temporary Agencies

Temporary work is a good way to get a handle on the job market. Many agencies specialize in placing people in short-term healthcare jobs. Nurses, nurse's aides, and medical technicians are among the types of workers most in demand for temporary assignments. Temporary employment can increase your job skills, your knowledge of a particular field, and your chances of finding out about permanent positions. It can also get your name out there in the field as someone who is capable, responsible, and talented. Some temporary jobs can lead to permanent positions. Whether or not your temporary job becomes permanent, it is in your best interest to take it seriously and impress your supervisor and coworkers. You will build your skill sets, making you more qualified for other positions. Besides, your supervisor and coworkers are all potential networking contacts for helping you find permanent work.

Job Fairs

Most colleges and universities hold at least one job fair per year. Do not dismiss these, even if you have just started your schooling. Job fairs are not just for graduating seniors looking for employment, they also are useful for enhancing networking skills. You should always attend job fairs in business attire and bring along at least ten copies of your resume. Be prepared for brief on-the-spot screening interviews. Practice summarizing your goals, qualifications, and special skills until you have a comfortable two-to-three-minute pitch that sums up who you are, what you want, and what you can offer. Some employers may want you to complete an online screening interview at the job fair; others may want to schedule phone, online, or in-person interviews on the spot, so be prepared for that.

Many companies also hold job fairs in order to hire employees. These fairs, which take place about once a year, are often advertised in your local newspaper's classified sections.

Job Hotlines

Each city has its own job hotline, monitored by the state employment agency. You can call your local employment agency for the phone number of the hotline that offers daily lists of jobs in your area. For a list of job hotline numbers, check the most current National Job Hotline Directory either online or in the reference department of your local library. Some local radio stations also offer job information and hotlines.

NETWORKING YOUR WAY INTO A JOB

Networking is a great way to get your name out in the community and find prospective career opportunities. It opens doors you might have never known about and allows you to find a job with the help of a reference, which is almost always better than searching on your own. Employers are more likely to hire someone based on a current employee's suggestion (so long as the employee is trustworthy and regarded highly within the organization). Make networking a priority task of your job search. Read on to find out why.

What Is Networking?

Networking means calling and talking about jobs in your area of interest with friends, acquaintances, and even people you do not know, and asking for advice and support. If you would like to work as a physical therapy assistant, for example, get in touch with all the people you know who work in hospitals or private practices or who have friends or relatives in the field. Talk to your family, friends, counselors, former employers, and anyone else you can think of who may be aware of a suitable job opening. You may discover a job even before the job opening is advertised.

Make a list of everyone you know in the healthcare field. Send a friendly email or letter to everyone on the list. You may want to include your resume when writing to people who are in a position to help you, or you can call and ask for permission to send it. Think about how you can begin making yourself more attractive, useful, and helpful to employers. Use your evaluation and your informal interviewing skills when you network with others.

You never know what opportunity someone will be able to find for you. A relatively small percentage of job vacancies are advertised to the public; many employers look for employees by word of mouth. This is called the *hidden job market*. In today's competitive climate, successful candidates must pursue all possible outlets. Networking is at least as important as visiting the career planning center at your school and checking help wanted ads. You want to gain as much exposure as possible.

Establishing Good Contacts

When establishing a network, you need to consider all possible living, breathing human resources: family, friends (including neighbors and parents of classmates), school personnel (teachers, counselors, alumni, administrators), previous employment contacts (employers, coworkers, customers, competitors), professionals (doctors, dentists, practicing professionals in your field), and community (businesspeople, and members of clubs, associations, chambers of commerce, and religious groups). You also can use magazine articles, newspapers, or other general publicity to begin targeting people you would like to include in your network. It is in your best interest to consider all reasonable possibilities.

Make sure to get permission before you use a contact's name when you put him or her down as a reference for a potential employer. Do not simply assume your friend will recommend you. Once you have received the networking information, use your own ability to get the job. A registered nurse from Jackson, Mississippi, explains:

> *I asked my uncle, who was a surgeon at a local hospital, if he knew of any openings around his hospital. I had been working for a nursing home and really wanted to get into a hospital where I might have more opportunity for promotion. He said he would get back to me, and when he did, he gave me the name of the nursing recruiter. He had talked her into giving me an interview before I even filled out an application. The interview was a success, and so is my career in nursing.*

Making Contact

Contacting a whole list of people for favors can be nerve-racking. However, the key to succeeding as a networker—and avoiding a major case of networking nerves and negativism—lies in understanding that you are not merely asking for a giant favor. You are subtly empowering the other party to make a recommendation to his or her company or organization that will help it for the better. You know you will be a great asset and a stellar employee; if someone recommends you and you succeed, he or she will end up looking great as well.

When you contact someone, first identify yourself clearly. If a third party referred you to this person, identify not only yourself but your referral source as well. Then explain your job objectives and how you would like your contact to help you. Your contact's willingness to help you will depend largely on how your requests are couched. Keep your requests for help brief, conversational, and low key. Be sincere and respectful of their time.

- ▶ Ask contacts if it is a good time to talk for about ten minutes, and then ask them to share any information they have about openings pertinent to your job goals.
- ▶ Tell them you do not need an immediate answer, and ask if you can call them back or meet on a specific date convenient for them.
- ▶ Use phrases such as *if I can make an appointment to speak with you*, or *if we can meet for a few minutes, so I might get your thoughts and opinions about some job-search ideas I've been thinking about*, or *if I can drop in on you at work for a few minutes and pick your brain*, or *if I can have your advice on getting some exposure in the healthcare market*.
- ▶ Keep it light and pleasant. To make it all easier, recite what you plan to say before you make that important call.
- ▶ Last, but certainly not least, write a letter to thank your contacts for their time. Tell them you really appreciate their help and that you are grateful for their willingness to mention you to their colleagues. Thank them as well for any referrals they may have given you. Also let them know that you will keep them posted about what happens. Many contacts will be interested to know that their input helped you.

Expanding Your Contacts

It is all right to ask the people you contact for other referrals. Your contacts may call the referrals to prepare them for your call and to make sure they are willing to talk with you.

Do not be afraid to contact people directly, even if they are complete strangers. You are paying them a compliment by contacting them. People like to talk about themselves. And remember, everybody likes a good listener. You are empowering these people when you ask for their personal advice, information, and wisdom. It is safe to assume that most of these people were in your shoes at one time, starting out in the industry and reaching out to anyone and everyone who might be able to help. Everyone knows what it is like to hunt for a job and most people are more than willing to put themselves out for someone eager to enter their chosen field.

Organizing Your Contact List

You will need to keep track of your contacts. Keep their names in an Excel spreadsheet or other electronic database, a notebook or personal organizer, or on three-by-five index cards. The most important thing is to find a tracking system that is comfortable for you and that you will use. Set up your network file to include the following contact information:

- ▶ name of contact
- ▶ address and telephone number
- ▶ how you met this person
- ▶ occupation
- ▶ date last contacted
- ▶ conversation summary
- ▶ names of referrals
- ▶ date of thank-you letter
- ▶ other comments

Maintaining Your Contacts

Keep in touch. Check in with your contacts every month to let them know how your job hunt is progressing. Keeping visible will generate further job leads. The key to faster success in your networking efforts is follow-up.

Unfortunately, the majority of your follow-up efforts will not produce valuable new information or insights. But a timely follow-up can jog your contact's short-term memory and get results.

In addition to writing thank you notes, you can clip and send relevant articles or follow up on personal information shared in your conversation. Perhaps your contacts mentioned a ball game they went to or a type of music they like; if you mention this again, you are likely to stand out in their memory.

WRITING YOUR INQUIRY LETTER

The first impression you make on an employer is likely to be the written word, delivered either on paper via mail or electronically. Many times, employers decide whether or not to give you a personal interview based on the quality of your correspondence. Your potential employer is likely to equate a well-written cover or inquiry letter with good work habits and a sloppy one with bad work habits.

A query letter or cover letter is written to inquire about an open position. A good cover letter should be neat, clear, brief, and, most importantly, specific. It should be no more than three or four paragraphs long. You should send this letter to a specific person, either the personnel/human resources director or the person for whom you hope to work. If you do not know that person's name, check the company website or call the company and ask to whom you should write. Find out that person's preference for receiving queries via email or postal mail. Honoring that preference is the first step toward making a good impression.

Begin your letter by explaining why you are writing. Let the person know that you are inquiring about possible job openings at the company, that you are responding to an advertisement in a particular publication, or that someone recommended that you write. Your letter should introduce the information on your resume and call attention to your qualifications. Add information that shows you are suited for the job. Always thank the reader for his or her attention to your letter, and add that you look forward to hearing back soon. Use the following examples to help you draft a personalized cover letter.

135 Lariott Court

Tampa, FL 12345

January 23, 2010

Gary Johnson

Personnel Department

St. Joseph's Hospital

P.O. Box 1565

Clearwater, FL 12345

Dear Mr. Johnson:

   I am writing to inquire about openings for medical assistants in your hospital. I have read and heard many favorable things about your hospital, and I feel that this would be the perfect work environment for me. The fact that St. Joseph's Hospital is a small but rapidly growing hospital presents some interesting challenges, and I am very interested in an available position.

   I recently graduated from the medical technology assistant program at Med Tech Community College and received a certificate as a medical assistant. I have experience typing business correspondence and putting together statistical and financial reports, and I am familiar with many different types of forms, including inventory and tax forms. My typing speed is 65 wpm. I have experience with customer relations, including answering telephones, greeting clients, and answering questions the clients may have.

   I have hands-on experience with all major office equipment, including computers and photocopiers, and am proficient with a variety of word processing programs as well as Lotus 1-2-3 and Microsoft Excel.

I always have been interested in helping people as well as working with computers. When I entered the medical assistant program, I learned that I am a hard worker as well as a caring individual. My training also taught me how to work under pressure while remaining organized to meet deadlines.

Enclosed is my resume, and I would be free to meet with you at your convenience. Also, I can arrange for you to speak with my references if you would like. Thank you for your attention to my letter. I can be reached at 111-555-9898 or at the address above. I look forward to hearing from you.

Sincerely,

Emily J. Small
Enc: Resume

6895 Peabody Avenue
Dallas, TX 45768
February 2, 2010

Elizabeth Townsend
Personnel Manager
St. Mary's General Hospital
P.O. Box 54G
Dallas, TX 45769

Dear Ms. Townsend:

I am writing in response to your ad in the Sunday, September 15, 1997, Texas Journal and Constitution. The ad stated that you are looking for someone with experience as a radiologic technician. I am a recent graduate of Bryman College's radiologic technician program with an associate degree, and I am looking for just this type of employment.

(continues)

I have a good rapport with patients, doctors, and other technicians, but most importantly, I like being a radiologic technician and am completely dedicated to my work. I will work hard to make sure a job is completed well, and I do not require constant supervision or reassurance to keep me working hard.

If you need a radiologic technician who is good under pressure, experienced, and completely dedicated, I think we have something to talk about. I have the talent, the knowledge, and the skills needed to be a successful radiologic technician.

Enclosed is my resume, and I would be free to meet with you at your convenience. Thank you for your attention to my letter. I can be reached at 777-555-1323 or at the address above. I look forward to hearing from you.

Sincerely,

James T. Anderson

Enc: Resume

WRITING YOUR RESUME

The word resume derives from the French word *resumer*, meaning *to summarize*, and that is exactly what you will do with your resume: briefly outline your education, work experience, special abilities, and skills. A resume also may be called a personal profile or a personal data sheet. This summary can act as your introduction by mail, your calling card if you are applying in person, and as a convenient reference when you are filling out an application form or being interviewed. A resume is usually required for getting a job, and it can help you more than you think.

The purpose of a resume is to capture the interest of potential employers so they will call you for a personal interview. That means you want to highlight the following:

- ▶ objective
- ▶ education
- ▶ work experience

► employment history
► special skills
► related experience
► personal qualifications

Preparing a self-inventory first will help you write a resume by pinpointing the items that show your ability to do the job or jobs in which you are interested. Select only those facts that point out your relevant skills and experiences. At the top of your resume, put your name, address, e-mail address, and phone number. Then decide which items will be most interesting to the employer you plan to contact.

Objective

Under your name and address you should state your career objective—your reason for contacting the employer. Describe briefly the type of position for which you are applying. Do not be too specific if you plan to use the same resume with different applications. You may need to give a general career goal; then, in a cover letter, you can be more specific about the position you are seeking in the particular company you are contacting. Of course, if you have the flexibility of your own computer and printer, then it is best to tailor each resume to a specific position.

Education

When listing your educational background, start with your most recent training and work backward. Employers want to know your highest qualifications at a glance. For each educational experience, include dates attended, name and location of school, and degree or certificate earned. If you have advanced degrees (college and beyond), you need not include your high school and elementary school education. You can also include any honors you earned at the school, such as being placed on the dean's list or graduating *cum laude*.

Work Experience

Every interested employer will and should check your educational background and employment history carefully. Employers do not want to hire people who have falsified their resume in any way. Make sure to list only past employers with whom you had positive experiences. If you do not have any related work experience yet, find some way to connect summer jobs, volunteer work, or part-time jobs to your current goals. For instance, when applying for a managerial position, it is appropriate to mention your job as a manager at a restaurant. Or you can highlight your interaction with customers to show your skill in working with the public.

Special Skills

You may wish to include another section called *Skills*, *Related Experience*, or *Personal Qualifications*. Write down any skills you think may be useful in your future job. These might include:

▶ computer skills such as data entry, database management, spreadsheets, billing software, electronic health record (HER) and electronic medical record (EMR), software, EHR/EMR, electronic reporting, and the like
▶ supervisory experience
▶ fluency in languages other than English
▶ experience working with new technologies (be specific)
▶ any work-related continuing education you have completed

Ways to Organize Your Resume

You can organize your resume in different ways to highlight specific areas of experience. Since some people have work experience and others do not, the different styles enable you to organize your resume in the most advantageous manner.

The Chronological Resume

The most common resume format is chronological—you summarize your work experience year by year. Begin with your current or most recent employment and then work backward. For each job, list the name and location of the company for which you worked, the dates you were employed, and the position(s) you held. The order in which you present this information will depend on what you are trying to emphasize. If you want to call attention to the type or level of job you held, you should put the job title first. Be consistent. Summer employment or part-time work should be labeled as such, and you will need to specify the months in the dates of employment for positions you held for less than a year.

The Functional Resume

The functional resume emphasizes what you can do rather than what you have done. It is useful for people who have large gaps in their work history or who have relevant skills that would not be properly highlighted in a chronological listing of jobs. The functional resume concentrates on your qualifications—anything from familiarity with hospital procedures to organizational skills or managerial experience. You can mention specific jobs, but they are not the primary focus of this type of resume. This type of resume is useful if you have little work experience.

The Combination Resume

A combination of the chronological and functional resume may best highlight your skills. A combination resume allows you to present your skills as well as a chronological list of jobs you have held. You get the best of both resumes. This is an excellent choice if you have limited work experience and want to highlight specific skills.

SAMPLE CHRONOLOGICAL RESUME

JEAN THOMPSON
1234 Third Street
Kansas City, MO 64131
816-246-4510
JeanT@aol.com

OBJECTIVE
To obtain a medical assistant position.

EDUCATION
Medical assistant certificate, June 1997
12-week program
Tad Technical College, 7910 Troost Ave., Kansas City, MO 64131
GPA: 3.95
Great Lions High School, Kansas City, MO 64130
June 2009
GPA: 3.98

WORK EXPERIENCE
Candy striper, nurse aide volunteer, 2008–2009
St. Mary's Hospital, Kansas City, MO 64130
Served meals and helped patients eat, dress, and bathe.
Delivered messages and answered patient call bells.
Completed daily filing and answered telephones.
Inventoried, stored, and moved supplies.
Assistant evening manager, 2007–2008
King Seafood Restaurant, Kansas City, MO 64133
Waited on tables and greeted customers.
Took over arranging staff schedule.
Balanced register and deposited money.
Learned how to order food and soft drinks.
Managed personnel when manager was absent.

COMPUTER EXPERIENCE
Typing 65 wpm
Macintosh, PC, Microsoft Word, WordPerfect, Lotus 1-2-3, E-mail

HONORS AND AWARDS
Student of the Year, Tad Technical College, Kansas City, MO

ACTIVITIES
Volunteer at Meltrice's Nursing Home in Wilmington, MO, and at local food shelters.

REFERENCES
References furnished from Tad Technical College, Career Planning and Placement Office, Griffin Hall, Kansas City, MO 64131; 816-555-1231

SAMPLE FUNCTIONAL RESUME

JACK WOODSON

1234 Second Ave.

Jackson, MS 10908

601-555-9876

OBJECTIVE

To obtain a career as a nursing assistant.

VOLUNTEER NURSING ASSISTANT

Two years volunteer experience as nursing assistant in competitive hospital.

Performed typical nursing assistant duties.

Monitored patient status.

Became familiar with radiologic technology by taking bone x-rays.

CLINIC ASSISTANT

Assisted medical assistant with paperwork and filing.

Ran basic errands and answered phones.

EDUCATION

Associate degree in radiologic technology, June 2009

University of Mississippi Medical Center, Jackson, MS

Major: Radiology

GPA: 3.8/4.0

REFERENCES

References furnished by the Career Planning and Placement Center, University of Mississippi, Jackson, MS; 601-555-9876

SAMPLE COMBINATION RESUME

Jennifer Perkins
Dental Assistant
1234 Obart St.
Orlando, FL 33054
407-555-7656

OBJECTIVE
To obtain a position as a dental assistant.

QUALIFICATIONS
Skilled dental assistant. Good rapport with dentists and patients. Specialty in periodontics. Expertise in all areas of general practice dentistry. Knowledgeable in office procedures. Devoted to patient education.

EDUCATION
College of Medicine and Dentistry
University of North Carolina, Chapel Hill, NC
Dental assistant certification, 2008

CLINICAL TRAINING
Administrative training includes:
- Scheduling and confirming appointments.
- Sending and receiving faxes.
- Making orders for supplies and materials.
- Patient relations.

Clinical training includes:
- Knowledge of instruments.
- Preparation of tray setup.
- Providing postoperative instruction to patients.
- Removing sutures and excess cement.

RELATED EXPERIENCE
Volunteer dental assistant, West Front Free Clinic, Orlando, 1/07–12/08, assisting father's practice after school.
- Greeted patients.
- Filed insurance forms and treatment records.
- Scheduled and confirmed appointments.
- Answered telephones.

REFERENCES
Available upon request.

Resume Writing Tips

Employers and recruiters read countless numbers of resumes. Make your resume (and yourself) stand out by making it engaging, concise, and easy to read. The following tips will help you do exactly that.

▶ Print your resume in black on white, cream, or soft gray paper. Use matching envelopes.

▶ Put your full name and contact information at the top of the resume. Include your phone number, cell phone number, and e-mail address. Keep in mind that potential employers will form their first impressions of you from your resume. If your e-mail address contains racy, juvenile, or rude innuendo you may be passed over. Consider opening a new, free e-mail account to use specifically for your job search. Make your account address something neutral like your first initial and your last name, or your last name and zip code. Two of the many free e-mail options available to you on the web are www.yahoo.com and www.gmail.com.

▶ Use 11 or 12 point Arial or Times New Roman font.

▶ Include ample white space. Use 1.5- or double-spacing and 1-inch margins.

▶ Proofread carefully, and use spell check and grammar check software if necessary.

▶ Use active language. Use words that highlight your energy and initiative, such as *initiated, developed, created, fostered, cross-trained, sought,* and *partnered.*

▶ Be consistent in writing style and document formatting. Double-check spacing, bullets, headings, bold face, and font to ensure consistency throughout your resume.

▶ Be positive and confident in your resume, but never lie or embellish. Demonstrate to employers that it is worth their time to interview you.

▶ If at all possible, limit your resume to one page. While it is better to go to two pages than to crowd your information, having a one-page resume as your goal will keep you focused and concise.

▶ Go to your local library or bookstore, or access online resources to read more sample resumes.

ACING YOUR INTERVIEW

The interview is the most important aspect of a job hunt. The first impression you make on a prospective employer could be the reason you do or do not get the job. Many employers conduct screening interviews, which are a way for employers to eliminate candidates who are clearly unqualified. If you have completed the necessary education and training, and can highlight your relevant qualifications, you should not have any difficulty with screening interviews. Whether online or on the phone, it will be helpful for you to have a copy of your current resume on hand during the screening interview.

Some employers utilize personality profiles throughout the interview process. Again, these may be conducted online, on the phone, or face to face. Candidates must achieve a certain score on the personality profile in order to advance to the next phase of the interview process. It is most important to answer the questions honestly. Employers look for different types of people at different times, depending on their needs. If you are not advanced to the next interview phase it may mean that although you have the skills for the job, you are not the best fit. Stay positive. It would not do you any good to accept a job that is not well suited to your personality. Interviewing is about finding the right fit for both employer and employee.

Many people are nervous about interviews, but know that being well prepared can lessen your anxiety. Interviewers are looking for specific qualities when they ask questions. In addition to probing your knowledge, they are observing how you organize your thoughts and how you communicate. Breathe. Compose your thoughts. Be yourself.

Informational Interview

Arrange an informational interview with someone who is in a position similar to the one you want. To make maximum use of the time that person is willing to spend with you, be sure to ask direct, pertinent questions and get complete information. This will enable you to make a better decision about whether to pursue a particular field. Here is a list of questions that will help you get what you want out of an informational interview:

▶ Please give me a general description of the work you do.
▶ What is your typical workday like?

▶ What do you find most rewarding about your work?

▶ What are the toughest problems you encounter in your job?

▶ What are the frustrations in your work?

▶ What compromises are most difficult to make?

▶ If you could change your job in some way, what would it be?

▶ What educational degrees, licenses, or other credentials are required for entry and advancement in your kind of work? Which are preferred or most helpful?

▶ What trade/professional groups do you belong to, and which do you find most beneficial in your work? Do any of them assist students interested in entry-level positions in your field?

▶ What abilities, interests, values, and personality characteristics are important for effectiveness and satisfaction in your field?

▶ How do people usually learn about job openings in your field?

▶ What types of employers, other than your own, hire people to perform the type of work you do?

▶ Do you know of any that offer entry-level training programs or opportunities?

▶ If you were hiring someone for an entry-level position in your field, what would be the critical factors influencing your choice of one candidate over another?

▶ Is there anything else you think I would benefit from knowing about this field?

After an informational interview, not only will you be more knowledgeable about your prospective position, but you also will gain interview experience, which may lessen your anxiety when it comes to the actual job interview.

Preparing for Your Interview

Preparation will enable you to be confident, overcome interviewing inexperience, and sell yourself and your qualifications. You should have a few clean copies of your resume with you (even though the company may already have it, it makes a great impression if they need an extra copy and you have one ready) as well as a personal inventory (a reference of possible answers to interview questions) to guide you as you describe your strengths and give examples to support your resume. One way to create a personal inventory is to write a short personal autobiography. Having this small autobiography handy will help you remember answers to the more challenging interview questions.

Research the company you are applying to so you feel more comfortable and can demonstrate genuine interest in the company during the interview. The public library is a good source for this kind of information, as are health publications. The idea is to converse knowledgeably about the company during the interview.

Dress for success. This may seem trivial, but you would not want to miss a job opportunity simply because of unprofessional attire. What you wear says a lot about your personality and attitude. Dress to show you are proud of yourself and your accomplishments. Even if you know that the institution dress code is business casual, you should be in business dress. For men, a conservative suit with a white shirt and contrasting tie, well-shined shoes, and socks over the calf should be appropriate. For women, a jacket and skirt or dress in navy or black, neutral or sheer hose, simple pumps, and simple makeup are appropriate for most situations. Avoid distracting styles and accessories, like dangling earrings and neon-colored ties.

Allow sufficient time for the interview. You will likely be interviewing with more than one person during the interview cycle. You will not be at your best if you are worried about another appointment. It is a mistake to rush your interviewers because you have made a previous and conflicting commitment for the same day.

Arrive at the interview early. Arriving on time shows your respect for the interviewer and your professionalism. You do not want to be late. Allow extra travel time if you are unfamiliar with the employer's location.

Keep yourself in a positive frame of mind. Remember that you are there to discuss job-related topics, not your personal problems. If your interview begins on a negative note, it may be difficult to turn the atmosphere around later. Begin with a positive attitude.

Go to the interview alone. If your spouse or a friend takes you to the interview, have that person wait for you elsewhere. A third party can be a negative distraction for both you and the interviewer.

Answering Tough Interview Questions

Employers tend to ask potential employees two kinds of questions: directive and open-ended. Directive questions attempt to gain, clarify, or verify factual information. Application forms are a series of directive questions. *Where did you go to school? How long have you worked as a radiologic technician?* and *What are your salary requirements?* are all directive questions.

The open-ended question is an effort to draw out strengths and weaknesses. Many employers conduct a *behavioral* or *situational interview*. They will ask you to describe a variety of challenging situations, for example, *Tell me about a time when you made a decision that was unpopular with your peers* or *Tell me about a time when you accomplished something very significant*. In asking these questions employers want to learn three things:

1. What was the challenge or problem?
2. What did you do about it?
3. What was the outcome of your actions?

To keep your response focused on those three things, choose situations that demonstrate your ability to solve problems and that show a clear connection between your actions and a positive resolution. Honesty and integrity are extremely important in the healthcare industry. It will be helpful if you can describe a situation that highlights your integrity.

Some employers also may ask illegally discriminatory questions, probing for information that will lead them to draw conclusions based on stereotypes or assumptions about human behavior. It is illegal for employers to ask certain direct questions about your personal life, such as your age or whether you are married or have children. However, employers may legally ask questions about your ability to fully discharge all responsibilities of the job for which you are applying. For example, if you are asked whether there is any reason you would not be able to work nights and weekends, you can simply answer Yes or No or you can indicate that you have young children or some other commitment that would interfere with that type of schedule. If you share personal information during the interview, the employer is then at liberty to talk with you about that personal information. However, you always reserve the right not to answer any question you feel is inappropriate.

To deal effectively with all types of interview questions, you need to consider the employer's point of view. No matter what kind of question is asked, an employer really has only four questions:

1. Can you do the work? (Do you have the skills, competence, and credentials?)
2. Will you do the work? (Do you have the motivation and stamina to produce?)
3. How well will you really be able to do the work?
4. Can you get along with others, especially with me, your supervisor? (What are your interpersonal skills and key personality traits?)

A hospital employment manager from Jacksonville, Florida, describes a typical interview at her hospital:

> *At our hospital, we give what is called a pattern interview, which is basically trying to find out how a person has acted in previous situations, whether at a job or in life situations, so we can find out how they will react in future situations. For example, I would say, "Tell me the best type of supervisor that you could work under" or "If you were caught in an error, how did you respond to that and solve the problem?" Most people will tell you exactly what they've done in the past, which is a good indication of what they will do in the future. We do not ask hypothetical questions. We want to know what they've done in reality.*

When responding to questions, ask yourself: What is the underlying question? This is particularly important with open-ended and discriminatory questions. Accuracy and specificity are the keys to directive questions. The ability to understand yourself as a product and to express your strengths will help you answer open-ended questions more effectively.

Here are some questions frequently asked by employers:

- ► Tell me a little about yourself.
- ► Why should we hire you?
- ► What are your career objectives?
- ► If you could have the perfect position, what would it be?
- ► Do you have plans for continuing education?

- ▶ Why did you choose this career field?
- ▶ In what type of position are you most interested?
- ▶ What do you expect to be doing in five years?
- ▶ What is your previous work experience? What have you gained or learned from it?
- ▶ Why are you interested in our organization and in this particular opening?
- ▶ What salary do you expect to be earning now? In five years?
- ▶ Why did you choose your particular course of study?
- ▶ What do you consider to be your major weaknesses? Strengths?
- ▶ In what ways do you think you can make a contribution to our organization?
- ▶ What two or three accomplishments have given you the most satisfaction?
- ▶ Describe your most rewarding college experience.
- ▶ What have you learned from participation in extracurricular activities?
- ▶ Are you willing to relocate? Are you willing to travel?
- ▶ Do you think your grades are a good indication of your academic achievement?
- ▶ What have you done to show initiative and willingness to work?
- ▶ What types of books have you read? What journals do you subscribe to?
- ▶ What jobs have you enjoyed most? Least? Why?
- ▶ What do you think determines an employee's progress in a good company?
- ▶ What qualifications make you feel you will be successful in your field?

Asking Questions

Frequently, toward the close of the interview, the interviewer will give you the opportunity to ask questions. Never say that you have no questions. This is your chance to set yourself apart from the competition. Prepare your questions in advance. Ask the most important questions first in case there is not enough time to ask all of them. Do not ask questions that might reveal a lack of research. It is inappropriate to ask about salary and benefits unless the employer is offering a position. Most employers do not want to discuss those issues until they are certain you are the right person for the job. Suitable questions include:

- ▶ What kind of career opportunities are currently available for my level of training and skills?
- ▶ Identify typical career paths based on past records. What is the realistic time frame for advancement?
- ▶ How is an employee evaluated and promoted? Is it company policy to promote from within?
- ▶ What is the retention rate for people in the position for which I am interviewing?
- ▶ Describe the typical first-year assignments.
- ▶ Tell me about your initial and future training programs.
- ▶ What are the challenging facets of the job?
- ▶ What are the opportunities for personal growth?
- ▶ What are the company's plans for future growth?
- ▶ What is the company's record of employment stability?
- ▶ What makes your practice different from that of your competitors?
- ▶ What are the company's strengths and weaknesses?
- ▶ How would you describe your company's personality and management style?

Follow-Up Protocol

Send a courtesy letter to thank the interviewer for his or her time. Mention the time and date of the original interview and any important points discussed. Mention important qualifications that you may have omitted in the interview, and reiterate your interest in the job.

Do not be discouraged if a definite offer is not made at the interview, or if a specific salary is not discussed. The interviewer will usually communicate with her or his office staff or interview other applicants before making an offer. Generally, a decision is reached within a few weeks. Show your commitment to their timetable. If you do not hear from an employer within the time suggested during the interview, follow up with a telephone call, but do not make a nuisance of yourself by calling every day for an answer.

THE INSIDE TRACK

Who:	Darren Denton
What:	Registered nurse
How long:	Over one year
How much:	$46,000 annually
Degree:	Associate degree in applied science in nursing
School:	East Tennessee University

INSIDER'S ADVICE

I began my career as a certified nursing assistant (CNA), the basic entry-level position after I completed a brief class. Then I went back to school to become a licensed practical nurse (LPN). I went back to school to get my RN degree and worked full time as well. I just slipped into a higher position once I received my associate degree.

When I first applied for the CNA and the LPN jobs, I had to undergo a complete physical, including blood work. I also had to submit a urine specimen for drug testing. I submitted an application and underwent two interviews for the job as an LPN. I then had to submit a resume and another application to advance to the supervisory position.

The worst part of the process was the interviews. I think everyone should take a class in interview skills, possibly a required high school course. If you get the chance to take a class, do it. You probably will feel more secure during the interview.

INSIDER'S FUTURE

I have set some long-term goals for myself. These include going back to school. I plan to obtain my bachelor of science in nursing degree (BSN) and then my masters degree in extracorporeal perfusion therapy (ECPT) to become what is known as a perfusionist in the medical community. The perfusionist is the person who, among other things, runs the heart-lung bypass machine during open-heart surgery.

CHAPTER six

HOW TO SUCCEED ONCE YOU HAVE LANDED THE JOB

THIS CHAPTER tells you how to thrive in your new career position. You will learn about managing work relationships, fitting into the workplace culture, managing your time, finding a mentor, and promoting yourself from within the workplace. Also, you will find interviews and helpful advice from employment supervisors and workers who are already in the field.

LANDING THE job is one thing. Keeping the job is another altogether. Completing a training program helps you understand work relationships, manage your time, and fit in, but when you are on the job as an actual part- or full-time employee, new challenges arise. Read on for useful advice on how to fit into the workplace culture, manage your time, and get along with your boss.

FITTING INTO THE WORKPLACE CULTURE

Many people are anxious on their first day of work, not only about whether they have the technical skill required to do the job, but also whether they will be accepted socially. The good news is that there are practical steps for fitting in and becoming a valued member of the team.

Most of these steps are grounded in common sense. Good rules of thumb include:

▶ Be on time for work and meetings.

▶ Restrict your personal phone calls at work.

▶ Strike a balance of formality—be neither too familiar nor too standoffish.

▶ Follow the rules of good ethics: take responsibility for your actions, do not take credit for someone else's ideas, and own up to your mistakes.

▶ Concentrate on your work rather than on the impression you are making.

▶ If you do not know something, ask someone.

▶ Do not be offended if coworkers do not warmly include you on the first day.

▶ Help your coworkers if they need it.

How easily you adjust may depend on the type of job and the size of the company, as Mindy Reynolds, a chiropractic assistant from Kansas City, Missouri, explains:

> *Being the newcomer can be hard, especially if the office is small and everyone has been there for a while. There were only six employees and two doctors at our practice when I first started. I just tried to be myself. I let everyone know that I had little experience other than training and that I would appreciate any help or advice that they had to offer. I was very open-minded and receptive to all the information everyone gave me. I also asked a lot of questions and wrote down everything I thought I needed to remember. You want to make sure you can get along with the others and carry on conversations about your job and life.*

Many institutions give new employees an orientation to make sure they understand the daily routine, such as where to park, office or work hours, and all basic policies and procedures. A general orientation may cover just about everything related to the company. In a department orientation, the resource person will work with new employees until they become familiar with their jobs. The length of such an orientation depends on employees' experience.

A department orientation is also an opportunity for you to become familiar with the interpersonal norms and culture of the institution. Here are some things you can do to become comfortable quickly in your new environment:

▶ Observe where and how work areas are arranged. Is there one community area in the center surrounded by smaller individual work stations? Do employees share all work areas? Do you see personal effects (such as pictures, notes, or plants) displayed anywhere, or is it all work related?

▶ Notice how employees address each other. Who is called by their first name and who is addressed with a title?

▶ Pay attention to the department atmosphere. Does it seem like a beehive, with everyone bustling around in high gear, or is the pace more relaxed? Do employees make time for brief social comments in between their work tasks? Do you see employees working together on tasks, or does it seem that people keep to themselves and their own specific tasks? Keep in mind that the work vibe may vary with the time of day, the day of the week, or the time of the year.

▶ Refrain from asking questions that may give the wrong impression of your work ethic. For example, asking *When do we get to break for coffee?* or *What is the procedure for requesting time off?* may give the impression that you have already decided you do not want to work hard.

Many hospitals or large institutions give helpful classes in areas such as time management, getting along with coworkers, and dealing with ethical issues. Your supervisor can sign you up, or you can sign yourself up, depending on your company's policy. Classes like these are becoming more and more popular in our complex, competitive society.

MANAGING WORK RELATIONSHIPS

Managing work relationships becomes difficult when people develop problematic behaviors. Many healthcare organizations rely on their employees to get along; when treating patients, employees cannot neglect their responsibilities or work on something else simply because they do not want to work with a specific person. Healthcare work is inherently a team process.

Managing your work relationships increases your own productivity. By learning about other departments and how other people's jobs rely on your work and output, you gain awareness of yourself as an important part of a larger whole. That can keep you focused and motivated when your work becomes routine. Exchanging information with people in other departments also expands your skill set and networking opportunities. You may learn about job openings in other departments, and having established relationships within departments outside of your own may make it easier for you to make a career move if one day you decide you would like a change. People are generally more willing to make an extra effort for people they know and like. Therefore, building positive relationships with people in the workplace can create a more efficient, productive, and stimulating environment for you and your coworkers and can open doors you might not have even thought you were interested in.

Aimee Davidson, a dental assistant from Huntersville, North Carolina, explains the importance of managing work relationships in her office:

> *As a dental assistant, I sit only about a foot and a half away from the doctor for almost eight hours a day. You want to make sure you can get along and that you can carry on a conversation without butting heads. You also want to make sure you know your job, so you won't slow the procedure down. You definitely have to be able to do several things at once and stay one step ahead of what the doctor wants. Doctors do not need someone who cannot get along with them or who doesn't know the job well.*

Here are some tips on building work relationships:

- ▶ Show integrity; demonstrate that what you say and do can be depended on.
- ▶ Be efficient. Do not blatantly waste time. The longer you take to get things done, the more repercussions your colleagues will feel. People know when you are being slower than normal because you are being thorough (which is fine!) and when you are just being lazy.

▶ Show team spirit, especially if you are working with a team of people on a project.

▶ Demonstrate a good attitude.

▶ Complain with caution, both to peers and to your higher-ups. You never know who might be listening or to whom your colleagues might run to tell your each and every gripe. Try every other avenue to resolve conflict before complaining to your boss. Like tattling, it could backfire.

▶ Do not get too personal or ask intrusive questions.

▶ Do not tell everyone your life story or let them know you are having a bad day. When people ask *How are you?* they generally expect to hear *Fine*, not a report on your headache or your kidney stones.

▶ Keep personal work issues to yourself to prevent gossip. If you have a problem, go to your supervisor and discuss it. Do not ignore the problem and expect it to work itself out, or you may be labeled the problem maker.

▶ Do not use any obscene or discriminatory language or make jokes that someone else might find offensive. This is especially true because you are surrounded not only by peers but also by patients.

▶ Do not expect everyone to be your best friend, or even as helpful as you would like or expect them to be. Some people take their jobs more seriously than others' jobs. Others are not, by nature, cooperative and willing to sacrifice their time to help their colleagues. Although in a perfect work environment everyone would work together and help each other out, do not expect everyone to take time out for you.

▶ Sincerely thank everyone who does help you.

If you do your job correctly and efficiently, mind your own business, and maintain a positive attitude, no one will be able to find fault with you as an employee. Cathy Holmes, a hospital unit secretary from Tampa, Florida, says:

> *When I began in the hospital, most people were friendly and helpful. Do not be afraid to ask for help from others. Try to get along with the people you work with. Know that there are differences in personalities and lifestyles. Remember that you do not have to socialize outside the workplace. And do not gossip—you never know who may hear what you are saying.*

Additional Success Tips

- ▶ Make an effort to show up for work on time, all the time.
- ▶ Show enthusiasm for new projects.
- ▶ Smile and greet your supervisors when you meet them in the hall.
- ▶ Be honest.
- ▶ Refrain from gossip.
- ▶ Do not be afraid to ask for help, and do not automatically think you know everything.
- ▶ Keep a positive attitude to create a positive atmosphere.

TIME MANAGEMENT CHALLENGES

Efficiency is key for success in any office job. You need to manage your time wisely so as not to get bogged down by your workload or appear unable to handle your job. Many factors can make you inefficient on the job. Here are some culprits to watch out for as your navigate the waters of a new job. (Look for time management solutions in the next section.)

Disorganization

Your inefficiency may spring from basic disorganization of workspace and time. If you find that you often stay late or leave unfinished work, or feel there are not enough hours in the day, disorganization may be to blame. Taking too many breaks, socializing, and procrastinating are often at the root of the problem. Change these habits and attitudes, and becoming organized will be easier. Lack of motivation can contribute to time management challenges as well, and may signal a desire for more responsibility or a job change. If this is the case, talk to your supervisor about taking on tasks outside of your normal job description. If you accept more responsibility and still manage to thrive, you will quickly catch the eye of higher-ups in your place of employment, which can lead to promotions and glowing recommendations.

Procrastination

Procrastination may look like disorganization because in both cases you end up finishing tasks late, but the two problems are not the same. Procrastination springs from one of three main sources: basic dislike of and lack of commitment to the task at hand, fear of not being able to measure up, or perfectionism. Like distraction, procrastination may be a sign that you are ready for a more challenging position.

Distraction from Outside Sources

If you have too many distractions, you will find it hard to finish tasks or even to leave work on time. Distractions lead to a loss of concentration that can spell disaster for your workday. And in the healthcare world, not completing tasks affects others besides yourself. For example, if you are a nursing assistant and have not finished your tasks before leaving, the assistants who come in after you are not going to be happy about having to do your leftover work. The work in this industry is such that it has to get done within a certain time frame—work left undone by you is often work that someone else must then complete for you. Too much socializing, a cluttered workspace, and a constant flow of traffic by your station or desk can all affect your ability to concentrate. If you cannot move your work station to a quieter place, try to position your computer or paper work so that you face away from the traffic corridor when you are working.

Excessive On-the-Job Stress

On-the-job stress generally springs from two sources: internal pressure and external pressure. Often, the greatest pressure we have to bear is that which we put on ourselves. Internal pressure is pressure you put on yourself to perform well, to achieve your goals, to meet others' expectations, or to fit into a particular role. Some of it is necessary—it motivates you and drives you to get things done, and done well. However, it can reach bullying proportions and have the opposite effect if you let it. Following are three ways to relieve unreasonable pressure that plagues you from within:

1. Weed out unnecessary perfectionism—care more about overall excellence than minor details.
2. Care more about the quality of your work than about what others (including your boss) think of you.
3. Be nice to yourself.

Some people cannot stay awake, let alone work, unless they are constantly surrounded by hubbub and challenged by nearly impossible-to-meet deadlines that constantly loom on the horizon. Other people are distracted by the mere soft tap-tap of keystrokes at the next desk. Ask yourself honestly whether you work best in a busy office surrounded by other people, in a quiet office, or alone. If you are in an environment that is at odds with your personality or work style, you will likely feel excessive internal pressure. Often we have no choice: we have landed someplace and must make the best of our environment. Recognizing the source of your internal pressure will help you develop strategies to manage it, even if you are not in a position to make a change.

External pressure is pressure put on you by other people, usually a supervisor, but sometimes by coworkers or other peers. If the pressure is legitimate—for example, your supervisor is pressuring you to record your clinical notes thoroughly and accurately—do your best to meet the expectation and relieve the pressure. If you believe that you are being unfairly pressured, you will have to choose from several courses of action. See Dealing With Your Boss later in this chapter.

TIME MANAGEMENT SOLUTIONS

If you are going to become a nursing assistant or a medical assistant, you will have a variety of daily jobs, both administrative and patient-care oriented. They may include typing, filing, scheduling appointments, making beds, delivering messages, helping patients eat or dress, and taking temperatures. Always keep this in mind: *take on one task at a time*. If you repeat this to yourself, it will help you not to get bogged down or exhausted. Keeping up with your workload, task by task, will help you be more efficient.

A surgical technician notes:

> *Time management is very important when you are getting ready for surgery, conducting surgery, and then cleaning up after surgery. There are times when I know the doctors do not need me, before and after surgery, so this is when I stock a room, check my supplies, get procedure instruments ready, and list what needs to be done. During surgery you have to be on the ball, aware of what instrument the doctor needs and what others around you are doing. You have to be on top of your job and know others' jobs, or it could cost the patient his or her life. I never have time to stand around, unless it is break time.*

Here are some effective techniques for overcoming the obstacles to good time management.

Create a To-Do List or Agenda

Begin by creating a master or rolling to-do list. List specific things you need to accomplish and the dates by which you need to have them done. Then work backwards to break your list down into smaller support duties, and schedule yourself to perform these duties in order of importance or time required. For example, if you are a medical assistant at a doctor's office and you have to complete an internal audit of patient records, start with *audit patient records*, then list each of the smaller tasks that make up the audit. Decide which needs to be done soonest, and do it first. Then delete or cross it off your list.

Here are just a few of the many electronic time management tools you can find online:

www.mindtools.com
www.evernote.com
www.zhornsoftware.co.uk/stickies/
www.rememberthemilk.com

Use Little Chunks of Time

Time leaks away in droplets, but it can be maximized in the same way. If you have five minutes before lunch and you have just finished a report, there is no reason not to start another, even if you will not finish it until after you get back. Or you can return one e-mail. Or make a quick call to a patient, if that is on your list. Do anything but sit there staring at the clock. You will be amazed at what you can accomplish. More importantly, making the most of your time will improve your attitude, giving you a sense of control over your day.

Reward Yourself

If you are working on a big task that takes several days, allow yourself a movie or dinner out after you have finished several small chunks. If it is a small task, allow yourself a snack at your desk. Reward yourself for your accomplishments; this is a great motivation. Seek support and affirmation from coworkers, family, and friends, and offer the same to them when they need it.

Eat Properly, Exercise, and Get Enough Sleep

Surprisingly often, boredom and lack of productivity at work stem from poor health habits, both on and off the job. Getting enough sleep at night is probably the single most important step you can take to improve your work performance. When you are tired, everything is harder, and all you can think about is quitting time. If you have difficulty sleeping you can get practical advice from the National Sleep Foundation at www.sleep foundation.org. Skipping breakfast and eating junk food for lunch and dinner has a similar effect. A light, nutritious lunch, followed by a short walk, can greatly improve the quality of your workday afternoons. The time you spend preparing and packing nutritious snacks or meals will be time well spent.

Alternate Tasks to Add Variety

If you have some say in how you spend your time at work, add variety to your day by changing from one task to another rather than devoting a whole day to a single task. Try spending a little time typing, then some time filing, and then some time photocopying; this can stave off boredom and keep you from watching the clock. Besides, the more job tasks you master, the better your chances of advancement.

Take Mini-Breaks

Sitting in one place, in one position, for long periods can be stultifying. But suppose you have taken on a one-task job and do not have the luxury of moving about or alternating tasks. Taking unobtrusive mini-breaks will not only alleviate body strain but aid relaxation. Here are some simple mini-breaks:

- ▶ Stand up and stretch a moment, then sit back down.
- ▶ Yawn and blink (these also help release tension and lubricate eyes).
- ▶ Massage your hands and fingers or cover your eyes with your palms.
- ▶ Do deep breathing exercises in your seat.
- ▶ Do isometric exercises, such as calf flexes, ankle twirls, stomach tightening and relaxation, gentle shoulder shrugs, and head-rolling.
- ▶ Stretch while remaining seated; clasp your hands behind your head and pull your elbows and shoulders way back (this is called the executive stretch).
- ▶ If allowed, get coffee or, better yet, juice or a healthy snack, and bring it back to your desk.
- ▶ Visit the bathroom once between breaks. Not even the strictest boss can fault you for that.

Rearrange Your Workstation

If you find yourself distracted by others—either because people tend to stop at your desk to chat or because they bump into your desk as they pass—it is best to reposition your workstation, if you are allowed to do so. You may want to turn so that you face a wall or window, or at least so you are not facing into oncoming traffic.

DEALING WITH YOUR SUPERVISOR

Your success is directly tied to the relationship you have with your supervisor. Your supervisor may direct scheduling, make all major assignments, set deadlines, and complete employee performance evaluations. If you do not get along with your supervisor, your preferences and interests may not be fully considered when making department decisions. Also, if you and your supervisor have a negative relationship, that can make it difficult for your supervisor to evaluate your performance objectively. You may not get the recognition you have earned or you may not receive strong support for advancement.

Some supervisors are supportive, encouraging, and objective. However, unfortunately, some are critical, demanding, and just plain unfair. If you have examined your heart and have come to the conclusion that your situation truly seems to be unpleasant, and that in fact you are working for a boss you find hard to tolerate, you have three options:

1. Accept the situation.
2. Find another job, then quit this one.
3. Work to change the situation. You can fight, but be prepared to pay a heavy price unless you have a good union. You can seek mediation or counseling, either through the Employee Assistance Program (EAP) or outside your work.

Some supervisors are unintentionally difficult to work for. They operate under constant pressure, and that pressure is very likely to spill over onto you. If you are not sure whether your supervisor is unreasonable or just has high expectations, keep accurate records of meetings, e-mail messages, and phone calls. Save relevant memos, directives, and performance appraisals, and arrange to review them with an EAP counselor or another professional advisor.

If you decide to accept your supervisor as is, here are some key strategies for managing unreasonable external pressure:

▶ Remember that you have a life outside work. Strive to do your best work while at work, then leave it at work.

▶ Set limits, even with your boss. The EAP can offer guidance on when and how to communicate appropriately about this with your supervisor.

▶ Learn physical relaxation techniques. Yoga, deep breathing, and desk-side stretching can all help to relieve stress and restore your motivation.

FINDING A MENTOR

One of your best resources at work is a good mentor. Some institutions call them *resource persons*. A mentor or resource person can help you greatly while you learn about your new job, get acquainted with your new building, and begin to adjust to your work surroundings. He or she also may teach you things about your job that you did not learn in school.

Ronald Shane, an optometrist from Pennsylvania, describes his mentor:

> *I am most grateful that the chief of the eye department at Giselle became my mentor and good friend. I will always be indebted to Dr. Richard Appell for the knowledge he has given me, as well as his guidance and friendship. He has changed my ideas about what optometry should be. I graduated from optometry school knowing a great deal about the eye but having no concept of what "vision" is. Dr. Appell showed me the difference between acuity and vision.*

PROMOTING YOURSELF

Many times in your career you will have chances to promote yourself to a higher-level position or better hours. Before you ask for a promotion, show your employer or supervisor that you have dedicated yourself to your current position, that you have performed well, that your attendance is satisfactory, that you have been cooperative and flexible, and that you have gained the necessary training.

Hospitals usually hire entry-level workers for a contract position. You may be hired as a nurse's aide and required to keep that position for six months before requesting a promotion or a schedule change. You should only accept the job if you can commit to these terms. A nursing recruiter from Athens, Georgia, explains:

> We tell applicants, "These are the hours of this position. Is there anything that would prevent you from working these hours?" We have got to know if the person's going to be able to work the hours. Some people will say they want days but they'll take nights. Well, we try not to do that because when you are hired into a night position, you are committed to that, and a lot of times, those people start applying right away to change to days. You cannot do that. Do not take the job just to get your foot in the door.

After six months you are eligible to transfer if you have the qualifications and if your employment record is clean. You will need to fill out a job transfer request form explaining to your supervisor and others when and why you wish to transfer. You will not be promoted if you have performance or attendance problems.

Private practices and group practices hire different numbers of staff and have different work policies. You may be promoted as soon as you receive the training needed for a promotion, if the physician feels you can do the work. Here it is up to the employer; in hospitals, promotions follow more formal guidelines.

ACHIEVING SUCCESS

Once you have landed the job you have worked so hard to get, do your best to make it worth your time and energy. Commit yourself to doing your job well, and prove to your boss that you appreciate the chance to succeed. Find people in your work environment to take you under their wing. Identify the higher achievers in your department and make a point to spend time with them. Let them know you take your work seriously and would like to get better or move up, depending on your goals. Tell them that you admire their work and you appreciate any guidance they can give you. Some people will be flattered and will welcome the opportunity to help you; others will not want to be bothered. Do not take it personally; continue to be friendly and learn what you can just by observing them.

Form friendly relationships with coworkers, sharing ideas and common interests. It will make your work environment more enjoyable and help you stay motivated during stressful times.

Come to work on time, be efficient, and, even when you are having a bad day, be positive and be careful not to take it out on someone else.

Take classes in time management or work relationships if you need them. Promote yourself after you have proven your capabilities in a probationary period. Show everyone your best, and you will succeed and move on to greater opportunities and higher levels of pay.

THE INSIDE TRACK

Who:	Catherine A. Holmes
What:	Unit secretary II, surgery scheduling coordinator
Where:	University Community Hospital, Tampa, Florida
How long:	11 years
How much:	$21,000–$24,000 annually
Degree:	Computer terminal operator certificate (comparable to a medical assistant certificate)
School:	American Business Institute

INSIDER'S ADVICE

Never stop learning. My willingness to learn new tasks helped me promote myself within my job area. I cross-trained for other positions and met managers in those areas. This broadened my contacts and demonstrated my abilities and worth. If you prove to your supervisors that you want to be successful at the job you have and want to learn more about other positions as well, your supervisors will eventually respond to that and move you up and around.

INSIDER'S FUTURE

I always wanted to be a nurse, since I was a child. I always wanted to help people and feel that my help really made a difference. I like the fact that there are so many different types of nursing jobs and a need for nurses almost everywhere you may travel. I am currently enrolled in a two-year associate degree in nursing program. However, I hope eventually to receive my BSN and possibly take management courses as well. I hope in five years to be working as an RN.

Appendix

Professional Associations, Directories, Accrediting Agencies, Internships, Scholarships, Placement Services, and Military and Travel Healthcare Careers

PROFESSIONAL ASSOCIATIONS

DENTAL ASSISTANT

American Dental Assistants Association
35 E Wacker Dr., Ste. 1730
Chicago, IL 60601
312-541-1550
www.dentalassistant.org

American Dental Association
211 E Chicago Ave.
Chicago, IL 60611
312-440-2547
www.ada.org

MEDICAL ASSISTANT

American Association of Medical
   Assistants
20 N Wacker Dr., Ste. 1575
Chicago, IL 60606
312-899-1500
www.aama-ntl.org

American Medical Technologists
10700 W Higgins, Ste. 150
Rosemont, IL 60018
www.amt1.com

NURSING ASSISTANT

American Academy of Nurse Practitioners
P.O. Box 12846
Austin, TX 78711
512-442-4262
www.aanp.org

American Assembly for Men in Nursing
P.O. Box 130220
Birmingham, AL 35213
205-956-0146
www.amn.org

American Association for Long Term Care Nurses
10979 Reed Hartman Hwy, Ste. 215
Cincinnati, OH 45242
888-458-2687
www.ltcnursing.org

American Association of Colleges of Nursing
1 Dupont Cir. NW, Ste. 530
Washington, DC 20036
202-463-6930
www.aacn.nche.edu

American Association of Critical Care Nurses
101 Columbia
Aliso Viejo, CA 92656
949-362-2050
www.aacn.org

American Association of Nurse Anesthetists
222 S Prospect Ave.
Park Ridge, IL 60068
847-692-7050
www.aana.com

American Nurses Association
8515 Georgia Ave., Ste. 400
Silver Spring, MD 20910
301-628-5000
www.nursingworld.org

American Nurses Credentialing Center
800-284-2378
www.nursescredentialing.org

American Society of Plastic Surgical Nurses
7794 Grow Dr.
Pensacola, FL 32514
800-272-0136
www.aspsn.org

Association of Pediatric Hematology/ Oncology Nurses
4700 W Lake Ave.
Glenview, IL 60025
847-375-4724
www.apon.org

Association of periOperative Registered Nurses
2170 S Parker Rd., Ste. 400
Denver, CO 80231
800-755-2676
www.aorn.org

Association of Rehabilitation Nurses
4700 W Lake Ave.
Glenview, IL 60025
800-229-7530
www.rehabnurse.org

Canadian Nurses' Association
50 Driveway
Ottawa, ON, Canada K2P 1E2
800-361-8404
www.cna-nurses.ca.cna

Dermatology Nurses' Association
15000 Commerce Pkwy., Ste. C
Mt. Laurel, NJ 08054
www.dnanurse.org

Emergency Nurses' Association
915 Lee St.
Des Plaines, IL 60016
800-243-8362
www.ena.org

Minority Nurses
www.minoritynurse.com

**National Alaska Native American Indian
    Nurses Association**
www.nanainanurses.org

**National Association for Health Care
    Recruitment**
2501 Aerial Center Pkwy., Ste. 103
Morrisville, NC 27560
919-459-2167
www.nahcr.com

**National Association for Practical Nur[...]
    Education and Service, Inc.**
1940 Duke St., Ste. 200
Alexandria, VA 22314
703-933-1003
www.napnes.org

National Association of Hispanic Nurses
1455 Pennsylvania Ave., NW, Ste. 400
Washington, DC 20004
202-387-2477
www.thehispanicnurses.org

**National Association of School Nurses,
    Inc.**
8484 Georgia Ave., Ste. 420
Silver Spring, MD 20910
240-821-1130
www.nasn.org

National Black Nurses' Association, Inc.
8630 Fenton St., Ste. 330
Silver Spring, MD 20910
301-589-3200
www.nbna.org

National League for Nursing
61 Broadway, 33rd Fl.
New York, NY 10006
212-363-5555
www.nln.org

**National Network of Career Nursing
    Assistants**
www.cna-network.org

National Student Nurse Association

Box 1211

Waterville, ME 04901

Nursing Assistant Central

www.nursingassistantcentral.homestead.com

Nursing Assistant Resources on the Web

www.nursingassistants.net

PHYSICAL THERAPY ASSISTANT

American Academy of Physical Medicine and Rehabilitation

330 N Wabash Ave., Ste. 2500

Chicago, IL 60611

312-922-9366

www.aapmr.org

American Physical Therapy Association

1111 N Fairfax St.

Alexandria, VA 22314

800-999-2782

www.apta.org

National Rehabilitation Association

633 S Washington St.

Alexandria, VA 22314

703-836-0850

www.nationalrehab.org

RADIOLOGIC TECHNICIAN

American Healthcare Radiology Administrators

490B Boston Post Rd., Ste. 200

Sudbury, MA 01776

800-334-2472

www.ahraonline.org

American Radiological Nurses Association

8515 Georgia Ave., Ste. 400

Silver Spring, MD 20910

800-274-4262

www.geronurseonline.org

American Registry of Diagnostic Medical Sonographers

51 Monroe St.

Plaza E One

Rockville, MD 20850

800-541-9754

www.ardms.org

American Registry of Radiologic Technologists

1255 Northland Dr.

St. Paul, MN 55120

651-687-0048

www.arrt.org

American Society of Radiologic Technologists

15000 Central Ave. SE

Albuquerque, NM 87123

800-444-2778

www.asrt.org

Joint Review Committee on Education in Diagnostic Medical Sonography

2025 Woodlane Dr.

St. Paul, MN 55125

651-731-1582

www.jrcdms.org

Joint Review Committee on Education in Radiologic Technology
20 N. Wacker Dr., Ste. 2850
Chicago, IL 60606
312-704-5300
www.jrcert.org

Radiological Society of North America, Inc.
820 Jorie Blvd.
Oak Brook, IL 60523
800-381-6660
www.rsna.org

Society of Diagnostic Medical Sonographers
2745 Dallas Pkwy., Ste. 350
Plano, TX 75093
800-229-9506
www.sdms.org

SURGICAL TECHNICIAN

Accreditation Review Council on Education in Surgical Technology and Surgical Assisting
6 W Dry Creek Cir., Ste. 110
Littleton, CO 80120
303-694-9262
www.arcst.org

American Association of Surgical Assistants
www.surgicalassistant.org

Association of Surgical Technologists
6 W Dry Creek Cir., Ste. 110
Littleton, CO 80120
800-637-7433
www.ast.org

National Board of Surgical Technology and Surgical Assisting
6 W Dry Creek Cir., Ste. 100
Littleton, CO 80120
800-707-0057
www.nbstsa.org

GENERAL

American Health Care Association
1201 L St. NW
Washington, DC 20005
202-842-4444
www.ahca.org

American Hospital Association
1 N Franklin St.
Chicago, IL 60606
312-422-3000
www.aha.org

American Public Health Association
800 One St. NW
Washington, DC 20001
202-777-2742
www.apha.org

Association for the Care of Children's Health
7910 Woodmont Ave., Ste. 300
Bethesda, MD 20814
301-654-6549
www.php.com

National Council on Aging
1901 L St. NW, 4th Fl.
Washington, DC 20036
202-479-1200
www.ncoa.org

National Health Career Association

www.nhanow.com

National Rural Health Association

521 E 63rd St.

Kansas City, MO 64110

816-756-3140

www.ruralhealthweb.org

U.S. Department of Health and Human Services

200 Independence Ave. SW

Washington, DC 20201

202-245-6296

www.hhs.gov

DIRECTORIES

AHA Guide to the Health Care Field

American Hospital Association

1 N Franklin St.

Chicago, IL 60606

312-422-3000

www.aha.org

Hospitals, clinics, and other healthcare organizations.

Allied Health Education Directory

American Medical Association

515 N State St.

Chicago, IL 60654

800-621-8335

www.ama-assn.org

American Association of Homes and Services for the Aging

2519 Connecticut Ave. NW

Washington, DC 20008

202-783-2242

www.aahsa.org

The AAHSA publishes numerous resources in the field of aging services.

American Medical Group Association

1422 Duke St.

Alexandria, VA 22314

703-838-0033

www.amga.org

The AMGA publishes a directory of physicians' private medical practices, as well as educational materials and special reports.

National Adult Day Services Association

85 S Washington, Ste. 316

Seattle, WA 98104

877-745-1440

www.nadsa.org

Adult daycare centers and state associations.

Federation of American Hospitals

801 Pennsylvania Ave., NW, Ste. 245

Washington, DC 20004

202-624-1500

www.fah.org

Healthcare facilities nationwide.

Hospital Phone Book U.S. Directory

Service

2807 N Parham Rd., Ste. 200

Richmond, VA 23294

804-762-9600

www.douglaspublications.com

Hospitals.

ACCREDITING AGENCIES

Accrediting Bureau of Health Education

Schools

7777 Leesburg Pike, Ste. 314

North Falls Church, VA 22043

703-917-9503

www.abhes.org

Commission on Accreditation of Allied

Health Education Programs

1361 Park St.

Clearwater, FL 33756

727-210-2350

www.caahep.org

INTERNSHIPS

Action AIDS

1216 Arch St.

Philadelphia, PA 19107

215-981-0088

www.actionaids.org

American Cancer Society Internships

Manager of Student Programs

250 William St., NW

Atlanta, GA 30303

www.cancer.org

American National Red Cross

2025 E St., NW

Washington, DC 20006

202-303-5000

www.redcross.org

March of Dimes Birth Defects

Foundation

1275 Mamaroneck Ave.

White Plains, NY 10605

914-997-4488

www.marchofdimes.com

Leukemia & Lymphoma Society

1311 Mamaroneck Ave., Ste. 310

White Plains, NY 10605

800-955-4572

www.leukemia.org

SCHOLARSHIPS

American Association of Colleges of Nursing
www.accn.nche.edu

Dental Assisting Scholarship Program
ADA Endowment Fund and Assistance
211 E Chicago Ave.
Chicago, IL 60611
www.ada.org

Maxine Williams Scholarships
American Association of Medical Assistants Endowment
20 N Wacker Dr., Ste. 1575
Chicago, IL 60606
www.aama-ntl.org
www.scholarships.com

PLACEMENT SERVICES

American Public Health Association Job Placement Service
800 I St. NW
Washington, DC 20001
202-777-2742
www.apha.org

American School Health Association Placement Service
7263 State Rte. 43
P.O. Box 708
Kent, OH 44240
330-678-1601
www.ashaweb.org

Medical Placements Service
Englewood Harbor
716 Stewart St.
Englewood, FL 34223
800-276-2269
www.searchmedicaljobs.com

National Association of Personnel Services
153 Shawneehaw Ave., Ste. 108
Banner Elk, NC 28604
www.recruitinglife.com

National Association of Temporary Services
119 S Saint Asaph St.
Alexandria, VA 22314

Paramount Healthcare Placement Services
2570 Blvd. of the Generals, Ste. 220
Norristown, PA 19403
866-831-1391
www.paramountplacement.com

MILITARY AND TRAVEL HEALTHCARE CAREERS

Department of the Air Force Headquarters
U.S. Air Force Recruiting Service (ATC)
Randolph Air Force Base, TX 78150
www.airforce.com

Department of the Army, Headquarters,
 U.S. Army Recruiting Command
Fort Sheridan, IL 60037
www.goarmy.com

Department of the Navy, Navy Recruiting
 Command
4015 Wilson Blvd.
Arlington, VA 22203
www.navy.com

Peace Corps
806 Connecticut Ave. NW
Washington, DC 20525
www.peacecorps.gov

Project HOPE
255 Carter Hall Ln.
Millwood, VA 22646
800-544-4673
www.projecthope.org

American National Red Cross, National
 Headquarters
2025 E St. NW
Washington, DC 20006
202-303-5000
www.redcross.org

U.S. Public Health Service
1101 Wootton Pkwy., Plaza Level
Rockville, MD 20852
www.usphs.gov

World Health Organization
(Pan American Health Organization)
525 23rd St. NW
Washington, DC 20037
www.who.int